THE MANAGEMENT OF ACUTE PAIN

GILBERT PARK

and

BARBARA FULTON

Department of Anaesthesia
Addenbrooke's Hospital
Cambridge

Oxford   New York   Tokyo
OXFORD UNIVERSITY PRESS
1991

Oxford University Press, Walton Street, Oxford OX2 6DP

Oxford New York Toronto
Delhi Bombay Calcutta Madras Karachi
Petaling Jaya Singapore Hong Kong Tokyo
Nairobi Dar es Salaam Cape Town
Melbourne Auckland
and associated companies in
Berlin Ibadan

Oxford is a trade mark of Oxford University Press

Published in the United States
by Oxford University Press, New York

A catalogue record for this book is available from the British Library

Library of Congress Cataloging in Publication Data
Park, G.R. (Gilbert R.)
The management of acute pain / Gilbert Park and Barbara Fulton.
(Oxford medical publications)
Includes bibliographical references and index.
1. Analgesics. 2. Pain—Chemotherapy. 3. Analgesia. I. Fulton,
Barbara. II. Title. III. Series.
[DNLM: 1. Analgesics—therapeutic use. 2. Pain—drug therapy.
WL 704 P235m]   RM319.P37 1991   616'.0472—dc20   91-3391
ISBN 0-19-263016-4 (hbk.)   ISBN 0-19-263003-2 (pbk.)

Typeset by Downdell Ltd, Oxford
Printed and bound in Great Britain
by Bookcraft (Bath) Ltd
Midsomer Norton, Avon

OXFORD MEDICAL PUBLICATIONS

THE MANAGEMENT
OF ACUTE PAIN

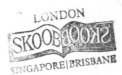

LONDON

SKOOB BOOKS

SINGAPORE | BRISBANE

Preface

The aim of this book is to provide simple practical guidance for those who prescribe and administer drugs for acute pain relief, particularly junior medical and nursing staff. This book is not intended as a comprehensive review of the subject or to replace current texts, but as a practical problem-orientated guide to an important subject which is often poorly understood and inadequately managed. Within the limits of this book's size, it is impossible to include every problem that may arise, but the information contained we hope provides a logical approach to any acute pain problem.

Drug dosages have been included for many drugs. Despite careful checking, mistakes may have occurred and if a dose appears incorrect it should be checked with the package insert, British National Formulary, or other suitable reference source, before the drug is administered.

We gratefully acknowledge the assistance and co-operation of the many medical and nursing staff, especially Mr P. Doyle, Dr M. J. Lindop, Sisters D. Pick and S. Bothamley, from whom we have received many helpful suggestions during the preparation of this book.

1991   B.F.
                                                            G.R.P.

Contents

1 Why is pain control a problem?

Numerous studies of hospital patients have confirmed that acute pain is often inadequately managed. Patients of all ages experience considerable pain during their hospital admissions despite the widespread availability of drugs and techniques to relieve pain. The reasons for ineffective pain control in hospitals have been a source of much speculation and study. Some of the major reasons which have been considered follow.

Lack of knowledge or interest in pain control

- Lack of understanding of the nature and pathophysiology of pain and methods of control.
- Lack of knowledge of the pharmacology of analgesic drugs and of alternative methods of administration available to improve drug efficacy can lead to inadequate prescriptions and poor analgesia.
- Lack of practical skill, not allowing regional analgesic techniques to be used.
- Lack of knowledge of adjuvant techniques and drugs to improve pain control.

Failure to assess pain, and its relief, accurately

The provision of analgesia is often dependent upon the assessment of a third party, nurse, or doctor. Judgements about the severity of pain may be made with no reference to the individual patient. One condition may be considered to be less painful than another and therefore less analgesia will be prescribed or administered.

There is often no review of the adequacy of pain control or the effectiveness of analgesic drug regimes. Prescriptions may be written but then there may be little follow-up of the effect on the individual patient.

Failure of communication

Patients must communicate their need for analgesia to the staff who are responsible for their care. There may be a number of reasons for a patient failing to communicate this need—not wanting to be seen to complain, the belief that it may be cowardly to need analgesia, or a simple lack of understanding of how to obtain analgesia. The ward staff also have a responsibility to communicate the facilities available for analgesia and how the patient may obtain help. Both sides may fail to communicate with each other.

Fear of addiction

Fear of addiction often leads medical and nursing staff to administer less analgesics to patients. Patients themselves may be concerned about this and consequently do not request sufficient drug to adequately control their pain. This fear frequently stems from a lack of knowledge of the true risks of addiction in patients who are receiving opioid drugs in the treatment of acute pain. *Addiction to opioids given for the management of acute pain is extremely rare*. It should not be used as an excuse for withholding opioid analgesics.

Fear of unwanted drug effects

The risks of unwanted effects such as respiratory depression with opioid drugs or gastrointestinal haemorrhage with non-steroidal anti-inflammatory drugs may often lead to inadequate drug administration.

Fear of masking physical signs

This problem may arise in a patient admitted as an emergency, where the fear of masking physical signs and making the diagnosis difficult is used as a reason for withholding analgesia. The patient with acute peritonitis may not be given analgesia—'until the surgeon has assessed him'. This is an unfounded fear. Analgesia *does not* mask physical signs.

The value of suffering

Some pain is expected as part of most illness or particularly after surgery and trauma. The goal of *no pain* is often seen as unachievable. Both patients and staff may have developed attitudes that associate suffering with self improvement—'Pain is good for you!' This is clearly not so.

Legal aspects of drug administration

Procedures for the administration of controlled drugs may often be inhibiting to staff and patients. Shortage of staff to check the drugs and fear of disciplinary actions if records are incorrect may add to delays and concern over the administration of opioid analgesics. In addition, the patient—appreciating the amount of work this means for nursing staff—may refrain from asking for analgesia.

A PRACTICAL APPROACH TO PROBLEM PAIN

This section is designed to introduce guidelines to the nurse or doctor involved in the management of patients in pain. Individual chapters of this book will deal in more detail with drugs and techniques that are mentioned here.

Treat the patient—not the symptom

Each patient is an individual. Pain control must be tailored to the patient's requirements. This begins with a careful evaluation of the whole patient, and requires frequent assessment of the individual patient's response to pain and its improvement with analgesics.

Pain should be treated according to what the patient feels and not what their attendants think they should feel. (see Beecher 1956*a,b*).

Individual variability

Drug response may be widely different between patients. The reasons for this are complex and poorly understood. The patient's response to an analgesic may also change with illness. Age-related changes have been documented—older patients may require less frequent analgesia than young patients. Standard prescriptions of analgesic drugs are therefore unhelpful and drug administration must be modified to suit the individual patient.

Choice of analgesic

Specific drugs may be useful in particular types of pain. In acute severe pain the standard drug is parenteral morphine, but mild to moderate pain may be treated with an oral opioid (for example dihydrocodeine) or a non-steroidal anti-inflammatory agent (such as ibuprofen). Choices may be modified by the patient's previous opioid exposure and current physiological and neurological state.

Pharmacology of drugs prescribed

It is important to have a knowledge of basic drug pharmacology. Factors such as the time of onset of drug action and the duration of analgesic effect are important considerations when prescribing analgesic drugs. How do the agents produce their analgesic effect? What are the unwanted effects associated with their use? All of these factors must be considered when prescribing analgesics.

Useful drug combinations

Opioid drugs administered in combination with non-steroidal anti-inflammatory drugs, antihistamines, or tricyclic antidepressant drugs can improve analgesic efficacy.

Administer analgesic drugs regularly

Infrequent intermittent administration of analgesic drugs will result in intervals of pain between doses. If this is combined with a prescription 'on demand' the patient must wait until pain is experienced before asking for further analgesia. Frequent regular doses of analgesic will go a considerable way towards improving pain control.

Use an appropriate route of administration

In acute severe pain the intravenous route should be used for the immediate control of pain once it has become established. Frequent intramuscular administration of analgesics gives effective analgesia and does not require the same technical skills and intravenous access. It may be a useful and practical method once the pain has been controlled with an intravenous bolus. Oral and rectal administration are more appropriate routes for providing prolonged analgesia in ambulant patients.

Use of local analgesic techniques

Useful techniques for providing analgesia using local anaesthetic agents are discussed in Chapters 13 and 14. The assistance of personnel skilled in the more complex techniques, such as thoracic epidural analgesia, may usually be sought from the department of anaesthesia, the intensive care unit, or from the pain control clinics that are becoming widely established in most hospitals.

Non-pharmacological techniques

Adjuvant psychological techniques such as relaxation and hypnosis may be appropriate in difficult patients. Assistance from interested and appropriately trained personnel will be required.

Careful monitoring and management of unwanted effects

This is mandatory whatever means are employed to treat acute pain. Staff involved in patient care must be well practised in patient resuscitation and in the recognition and treatment of the specific problems relating to drugs and techniques used to provide analgesia.

THE PAIN CONTROL LADDER

The concept of the ladder of pain control originated from the management of patients with chronic pain. However, it provides a

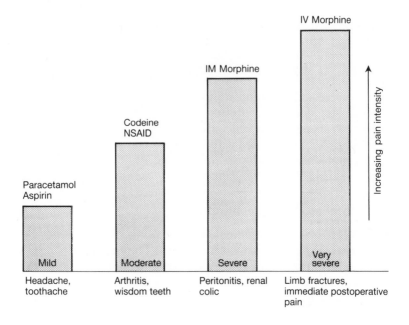

Fig. 1.1   A graphical representation of pain and analgesia

useful guideline for acute pain (see Fig. 1.1). Acute pain can be divided into mild, moderate, severe, and very severe. Any individual can be sited along this ladder of pain at any time. Patients with acute pain will tend to go down the ladder with time, as pain tends to decrease with time. This is unlike the patient with chronic pain from malignancy who may 'climb the ladder' as increasingly potent analgesics are required to control the worsening pain associated with the progression of the disease.

At the bottom of the ladder is 'minor' pain typified by a headache or toothache. This would usually be well controlled by oral drugs, most commonly the non-steroidal anti-inflammatory agents such as aspirin or paracetamol. Climbing the ladder, with pain of increasing severity, more potent analgesic drugs will be required. For moderate pain, oral drugs may still be sufficient and the oral opioids such as codeine may be used. In addition, the combination of oral opioids with aspirin and paracetamol are widely used. Such drugs would be helpful in the patient with pain following the extraction of wisdom teeth, for example.

Severe pain in the hospital setting is usually an indication for systemic administration of opioid drugs. Morphine is the standard opioid drug to which other agents are compared. Pain associated with trauma or after operation is commonly managed by intermittent doses of intramuscular opioids. Very severe pain immediately after operation, or in trauma patients after limb fractures, or breakthrough pain is best controlled by intravenous opioid analgesics to produce rapid improvement in analgesia.

2 What is pain?

Definition of pain

Pain is felt by all human beings on occasions. Usually it is of a minor nature (such as a headache or muscle strain) and usually it improves quickly without pharmacological intervention. Rarely it is severe, usually following injury or after a surgical operation, and may require intensive pharmacological efforts to relieve the pain and distress. Thus we are all familiar with what pain is and means individually. However, in scientific terms it has been defined by the International Association for the Study of Pain (IASP) as 'an unpleasant sensory and emotional experience associated with actual or potential tissue damage, or described in terms of such damage'.

A painful stimulus may be considered a protective response for the individual. Patients with diminished or altered pain sensitivity may develop severe joint injury and deformity and other damage because of the lack of pain sensation.

Physiology and neuropharmacology

Most pain originates when specific nerve endings are stimulated and nerve impulses are transmitted to the brain through the pain pathways. These receptors are known as nociceptors and can be divided into two types, described below.

1. Mechanoceptors

These are mainly present in the skin and respond to strong pressure applied to a wide area of skin and strong stimuli such as a pinprick and sudden application of heat (greater than 44 °C). They warn of potential damage and are the afferent part of the withdrawal reflexes. This type of receptor is associated with small myelinated primary afferent neurons designated Aδ (delta) type. These neurons transmit impulses rapidly. Stimulation of this type of receptor results in 'first' or 'rapid' pain which occurs early after injury and is usually sharp, localized, and pricking.

2. Polymodal nociceptors

These are the nerve endings of unmyelinated primary afferent neurons of the C type. They are widely distributed throughout most tissues and respond to tissue damage. The classification as polymodal indicates that they respond to tissue damage caused by mechanical, thermal, or chemical insults. In addition, they respond to chemical mediators formed or released as a result of tissue damage. These impulses are transmitted more slowly than impulses from the mechanoreceptors and travel along unmyelinated C-type nerve fibres. It is these impulses, from polymodal nociceptors, which are responsible for 'second' or 'slow' pain— slower in onset, prolonged, dull, aching, and poorly localized— after injury.

$A\delta$ nociceptors have a constant threshold below which stimuli are not perceived. For heat sensitivity this is about 44 °C. C fibres, on the other hand, respond to a range of stimuli of varying intensities and therefore have no minimum threshold value. It is the variation in the tolerance of pain at the level of the central nervous system (CNS), not the threshold at the periphery, which accounts for the wide variations in analgesic requirements of different patients. Thus two patients undergoing the same operative procedure may have widely differing analgesic requirements.

Both $A\delta$ and C fibres enter the spinal cord through the dorsal root where their cell bodies are located. After entering the spinal cord the majority of $A\delta$ and C fibres terminate superficially in the grey matter of the dorsal horn, which is arranged in a series of laminae. The $A\delta$ fibres terminate in lamina 1 and the C fibres immediately beneath them terminate in the substantia gelatinosa (lamina 2). It is in the spinal cord that the first 'processing' of painful stimuli occurs. The majority of both $A\delta$ and C fibres synapse either directly or, more frequently, via intermediate neurons in the deeper layers of the dorsal horn, with ascending fibres which cross the mid-line to join the spinothalamic tract. The details of synapses and connections in the dorsal horn are complex and beyond the scope of this book (for a review see Ottoson 1983).

Pain transmission can be inhibited at the spinal cord level by inhibitory interneurons or from descending inhibitory fibres. The best known theory describing how painful stimuli may be altered at the spinal level is the 'gate theory' put forward by Melzack and

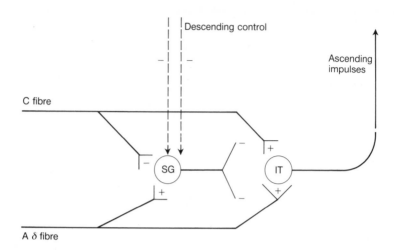

Fig. 2.1 A diagrammatic representation of the gate control at spinal cord level. SG, substantia gelatinosa cells; IT, intermediate transmission cells

Wall in 1965. They postulated that painful stimuli have to pass through a 'gate' in order to be relayed on to the central nervous system (see Fig. 2.1) This gate can be closed by non-painful sensory input carried by large myelinated fibres from mechano-receptors responding to low-threshold stimuli such as tactile stimuli, for example the immediate response of 'rubbing it better'. It is on this basis that transcutaneous electrical nerve stimulators (TENS) are thought to work. In TENS the mechano-receptors in the nerve distribution of a painful stimulus (for instance a surgical incision) are stimulated by a low-intensity electrical stimulation with the result that the gate is closed to the passage of the painful stimuli. In addition, the gate may be closed as a result of descending inhibitory systems; these originate in the periaqueductal grey matter and the descending tracts activate inhibitory interneurons of the enkephalinergic type in the dorsal horn (see Fig. 2.2).

In the dorsal horn of the spinal cord the principal neurotrans-mitter involved in pain transmission is thought to be the peptide, substance P, which is released in the dorsal horn after the stimu-lation of Aδ and C fibres. Opioid receptors are also present in the dorsal horn, particularly the substantia gelatinosa, and they are

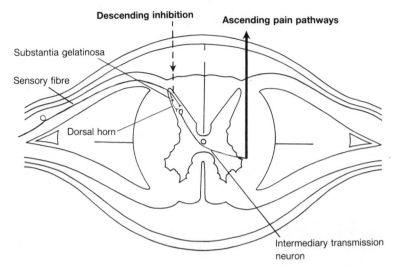

Fig. 2.2 The gate control—illustrated on a cross section through the spinal cord

thought to play an inhibitory role with enkephalins (endogenous opioid peptides) acting as neurotransmitters in the inhibitory interneurons.

Central pain pathways

Ascending pain impulses are transmitted mainly through the spinothalamic tract. Fibres from the dorsal horn project to lateral and medial areas of the thalamus from where further transmission of impulses is to areas of the sensory and motor cortex. This is the major route of sensory–discriminatory potential.

Ascending impulses may also travel via the spinoreticular tract and they do so more slowly, terminating in the pontomedullary reticular formation. These impulses have a major role in the arousal/motivational aspects of pain sensation, resulting from their connections with the limbic system. They are also respons-ible for the autonomic effects associated with pain resulting from the responses of the hypothalamus.

Descending pathways are mainly inhibitory in nature. Stimuli are produced in response to cortical and subcortical activation responding to sustained peripheral pain input. These descending impulses are visualized as controls over the 'gate'—thereby modulating pain input.

Neurotransmitters and pain

At the spinal cord level the principal neurotransmitter involved in the transmission of pain impulses is substance P. Other transmitters which have been identified include angiotensin II, somatostatin, cholecystokinin (CCK), enkephalins and dynorphins of the endogenous opioid peptides, 5-hydroxy tryptophan (5HT), and noradrenalin.

The chemical modulation of nociceptive impulses is complex. The place of agonist and antagonist drugs related to the neurotransmitters in the control of pain transmission is still undergoing evaluation. The hope that chemical modifications of the endogenous opioid peptides may lead to the development of an analgesic agent with few side effects remains the goal of many investigators in this area.

CLINICAL ASPECTS OF PAIN

Pain in some form will be treated by clinicians of almost every discipline. The varied causes of pain and the clinical settings with which it is associated may result in different perceptions of pain. As a consequence analgesic therapy may need to be adjusted accordingly.

Trauma

The assessment of pain in trauma victims shows that it varies greatly depending upon the cause. Often little pain may be felt at the time of injury; a soldier injured in battle or a fireman injured during the rescue of a child from a burning building may feel little immediate pain. However, the innocent civilian involved in a train crash or a bomb blast will complain of considerably more pain and may also require sedation because of the psychological and emotional shock of the incident.

The explanation of this phenomenon may be partly psychological—the need to get away from the cause of the injury overriding the pain and its immobilizing reflexes, and the need for involvement in the event for the soldier or fireman. In addition, pain and stress will also stimulate the release of endogenous opioids in the central nervous system, and these modify the pain response.

Early and effective analgesia is required after trauma, preferably at the scene of the accident, and it is not necessary to withhold reasonable doses of analgesics at this time while waiting for surgical assessment. Modern surgical assessment is less dependent upon the clinical signs—radiological techniques being widely available to aid in diagnosis. Pain itself may exacerbate shock and the most useful therapy at this time is small intravenous, bolus doses of opioid drugs. The only common exceptions to this include patients with a significant head injury and those suffering major blood loss, which may modify the need for analgesia or its amount.

Surgical pain

Adequate pain relief following surgery is essential for a rapid and uncomplicated recovery. The severity of postoperative pain is influenced by many factors. These are listed below.

1. *Site of operation.* Abdominal and thoracic surgical procedures are considerably more painful than peripheral and body-surface surgery.

2. *Time of day of surgery.* Morning operations are associated with less discomfort than those performed in the afternoon. This may be a result of diurnal variation in the concentrations of steroid hormones or modifications in the stress response to surgery. These effects may be mediated through the endogenous opioid peptide system.

3. *Sex differences.* The majority of studies of acute pain have demonstrated that female patients report higher *pain scores* than male patients after equivalent operations. However, other studies have shown no difference in *analgesic requirements* between the sexes.

4 *Previous pain experience*. There is a general expectation of pain after surgery. However, if patients have been in considerable pain from their illness or injury, which is relieved by surgery, postoperative pain may be less. Some patients with a background of chronic pain may experience more pain than would be expected after an acute injury or after surgery.

5. *Character of the pain*. Colicky, intermittent pain is less easily tolerated than continuous pain.

6. *Individual psychological factors*. These are discussed in Chapter 4.

Emergency surgery

The factors mentioned above will also apply to the patient who has just had emergency surgery, but there may be additional factors. Some of these are listed below.

1. Greater fear and anxiety may be aroused by the nature of the emergency. For example, after road traffic accidents the fear of blame may be a considerable concern that increases the emotional distress associated with the pain.

2. In some emergency situations the patient may have little or no time to worry, which may lessen the impact of pain.

3. Patients who have multiple injuries may have depression of their conscious level, which will decrease pain perception.

Non-traumatic pain

Patients with medical conditions unrelated to surgery or trauma may also suffer from acute pain and these illnesses similarly require appropriate analgesic therapy.

Myocardial infarction

The severe pain of myocardial infarction is an indication for opioid analgesia. Although modern research has concentrated upon methods of improving perfusion to the ischaemic myocardium with the use of intravenous thrombolytic agents and coronary angioplasty, the pain, distress, and anxiety that accompany the myocardial ischaemia will result in an increase in sympathetic tone and release of catecholamines. The accompanying tachycardia, dysrhythmias, hypertension, and increased myocardial work may worsen the ischaemia and hasten myocardial cell death. Thus the judicious use of opioid analgesics in these patients can improve cardiovascular function. The central effects of analgesics, by reducing the response to pain, will decrease sympathetic tone and catecholamine production. This, in turn, will result in reduction in the pre-load and after-load on the heart. When morphine is used the vasodilatation (probably resulting from histamine release) will further reduce myocardial work. However, in a few patients, after myocardial infarction analgesic agents may produce significant hypotension. The central mood-elevating effects of opioid drugs will also play an important role in alleviating anxiety in patients.

The choice of analgesic agent will depend upon the patient's level of pain, haemodynamic state, and respiratory stability, and how the drug may be expected to modify these parameters. Opioids are generally the standard agents and morphine and diamorphine the most widely prescribed. These should be administered intravenously; intramuscular administration may result in widespread bruising if the patient is receiving thrombolytic therapy.

Nausea and vomiting may counteract the benefits of the opioids so an appropriate antiemetic should be administered with them. Dysphoria may also be seen after the administration of some opioids and this may result in unwanted restlessness and agitation.

Inflammatory pain

Examples of acutely painful inflammatory conditions include acute pancreatitis and acute arthritis (rheumatoid, gout, etc.). The inflammatory process leads to the formation of tissue oedema which, with increasing tissue tension, results in pain. In addition, substances released during inflammation and cell damage, such as histamine, prostaglandins, substance P, 5-hydroxy tryptamine (5HT), and kinins sensitize the afferent nerve endings, making them more sensitive.

Opioid drugs may be needed to control severe pain from these causes. This type of pain may also benefit from non-steroidal anti-inflammatory drugs (NSAIDs) for both their analgesic and anti-inflammatory properties. Drugs such as indomethacin, diclofenac, piroxicam, and naproxen may be used in addition to opioids or on their own in less painful conditions. Acute gout is usually treated with high doses of NSAID.

Visceral pain

The differences in the transmission pathways of pain impulses from viscera result in pain of a different quality and character to that experienced from somatic pain resulting from other forms of injury. Visceral pain impulses are transmitted in fibres that are predominantly unmyelinated and found in sympathetic nerves. These can impinge on somatic input from the relevant dermatomes at spinal cord level and from there project to the brain in both the spinoreticular and spinothalamic tracts. There may be unpleasant discomfort, with or without pain, resulting from this, which is characteristically poorly localized.

THE ASSESSMENT OF PAIN

Pain is a sensation which is difficult to express and quantify. Further difficulties occur with its study since individual patients will react to similar painful stimuli in quite different ways, due to different perception and emotional response to the pain.

In some patients the cause of the pain will be immediately obvious (a trauma patient with a broken leg, for example), in others a complete history of the pain will be needed if it is to be adequately treated. The features that may be helpful in the diagnosis and assessment are shown in Table 2.1.

Once the pain has been characterized its severity can be evaluated. There are two approaches to the evaluation of pain severity (see below).

Subjective measurements

These rely mainly on the patients' expression of their pain. There are two basic methods available.

Table 2.1 Clinical features of pain used in diagnosis and assessment

Onset	Gradual, sudden
Main site	Chest, abdomen, limbs, wound pain, etc.
Radiation	Pain may also appear to radiate to distant areas from the principal site. The pain of angina pectoris for example typically radiates to the neck, jaw, and arm. Ureteric pain may radiate from the loin region into the groin. Hip pain may also be felt in the region of the knee
Character	Pain may occur in varying character and common descriptions include colicky, knife-like, constant, burning, etc.
Severity	Pain severity may be evaluated from the patients descriptive terms—awful, agony, unbearable, etc., or from specific questioning and appropriate rating scales (see text)
Duration	Minutes, hours, days
Aggravating factors	The pain of angina pectoris or intermittent claudication may be associated with exercise, whilst abdominal pain from peptic ulceration may have characteristic relationships to eating habits—aggravated by hunger and spicy foods. Pleuritic chest pain will be worsened with coughing and deep inspiration
Relieving factors	The patient may be aware of particular features that may ease the pain—a more comfortable posture, rest, etc.
Times of occurrence	Peptic ulcer may occur in the early hours of the morning; headaches related to raised intracranial pressure will occur in the mornings
Associated phenomena	Vomiting and visual disturbance may be associated with migraine headaches
Previous history	Of this or similar pain

Descriptive scales

These vary greatly in complexity but consist of a series of words describing pain severity from 'no pain' to 'severe'. An example of a simple scale suitable for clinical use is shown below.

1	No pain
2	Mild pain
3	Moderate pain
4	Severe pain.

Alternatively, to assess the effectiveness of therapy, a scale such as that shown below can be used.

1	No improvement
2	Slight improvement
3	Great improvement
4	No pain.

More complicated forms of descriptive scales are available as questionnaires, and these are primarily suitable for research purposes.

Visual analogue scale

This consists of a 10 cm line marked with a phrase such as 'no pain' on the left and 'the worst pain possible' on the right, as shown below.

No pain   -   The worst pain possible.

The patient is asked to draw a line through the scale indicating the severity of the pain. This can then be quantified by measuring the distance from the left of the scale. This is quick to use and relatively simple to understand. It can also be adapted for specific situations such as for children, when the words are exchanged for pictorial representations such as happy and sad faces. Visual analogue scales can also be easily computerized, the line appearing on a screen and the patient moving the cursor along it and the distance automatically measured.

Both descriptive scales and visual analogue scores are primarily designed to be used by patients but they can also both be used by an observer. However, this will considerably reduce the accuracy of the assessment. Subjective assessment can also be made, by an observer, of the physiological responses to pain such as pallor, sweating, and behavioural reactions.

Objective measurements

These are less frequently used than subjective methods as they are not always applicable and their sensitivity and reproducibility are limited. Many utilize physiological measurements which vary with the severity of pain. Most frequently these are respiratory measurements, which are useful measures after upper-abdominal and thoracic operations when pain may limit deep breathing and coughing. Such operations will be accompanied by reductions in arterial oxygen partial pressure, peak expiratory flow rate, and forced vital capacity, along with increases in arterial carbon dioxide partial pressure, and improvements may be correlated with adequate analgesia.

A further objective method of assessing pain is to record the patient's analgesic requirements. For example, to assess the effectiveness of a local anaesthetic block, the patient's opiate requirements before and after the block can be compared.

ENDOGENOUS OPIOID PEPTIDES

The discovery of the specific binding site for opioids in the brain in 1973 led the search to identify the endogenous chemical for which this was the receptor. In 1974 the first isolation of the enkephalins was announced and, the following year, the detection of β endorphin.

Opioid receptors

These high-affinity binding sites for opioids are located in high density in localized areas of the central nervous system. They are found in the dorsal horn of the spinal cord in the areas associated with the sensory processing of input from the C fibres and Aδ fibres that are important in pain transmission. They are also located in afferent vagal fibres. Although their function at this site is unknown they provide a useful experimental model for assessment of opioid-receptor binding. Large numbers of receptors are found in the limbic system and also in the hypothalamus in close relation to areas involved with neuro-endocrine control. Opiate receptors in the hypothalamus may be responsible for the release of antidiuretic hormone (ADH) or for the reduction in thyrotrophin-releasing hormone (TRH) and somatostatin and luteinizing-hormone-releasing hormone (LH-RH). They may also have important effects upon temperature regulation, the control over diurnal variation, and feeding behaviour.

Opioid receptors are also located in association with areas of both the parasympathetic and sympathetic divisions of the autonomic nervous system and these effects are useful as bioassays for opioid effects, although their functional significance remains unclear. Endogenous opioids act as neurotransmitters at specific synapses and may play a more widespread part as globally circulating hormones.

The following features suggest that the endogenous opioids identified are acting as neurotransmitters:

- they are actively synthesized in neurons;
- their presence in nerve terminals at synapses;
- they are released by depolarization of nerve terminals;
- endogenous opioids are rapidly inactivated by local aminopeptidases;
- they are present in high concentrations in specific areas of the central nervous system including the hypothalamus, pituitary, areas of the brain stem, and the limbic system;
- there are multiple stereo-specific structural analogues and antagonists.

Enkephalins

These are five-amino-acid peptides which have been classified as methionine or Met-enkephalin and leucine or Leu-enkephalin, depending on the N-terminal amino acid. They have an extensive distribution in the CNS and are found spinally and supraspinally.

β Endorphin

This is a 31-amino-acid peptide of which the sequence of the first five amino acids is identical to that of Met-enkephalin. This is an unusual opioid in that it has a limited distribution and is primarily restricted to a hypothalamic cell group.

Dynorphins

This is a third class of endogenous opioid peptides. The precursor peptide has three sequences each having a Leu-enkephalin core. Their actions are mainly at spinal cord level.

Endogenous opioid peptides appear to be mixed agonists with effects resulting from actions at more than one opioid-receptor sub-type. See Table 2.2.

Table 2.2 Classification of opioid receptors

Receptor	Effects	Agonist	Antagonist
μ(mu)	Supraspinal analgesia Respiratory depression Euphoria Physical dependence	Morphine β Endorphin	Naloxone Pentazocine
δ(delta)	Modulation of μ activity supraspinal analgesia	Leu-enkephalin β Endorphin ?Pentazocine	Naloxone Met-enkephalin
$\varkappa$(kappa)	Spinal analgesia Respiratory depression Sedation Miosis	Dynorphin Morphine Pentazocine Nalbuphine Butorphanol	Naloxone
σ(sigma)	Vasomotor stimulation Respiratory stimulation Hallucinations Dysphoria	?Not identified ?Pentazocine ?Ketamine ?Butorphanol	Naloxone

3 Why treat pain?

The most important reason for treating pain is a basic humanitarian concern; the first requirement of medicine being to alleviate suffering. Good analgesia will reduce patient discomfort and minimize the associated psychological distress. The role of analgesia in reducing morbidity after trauma and surgery remains unproven. However, the beneficial effects seen on several organ systems as a result of improved pain control may lead to improved outcome and a reduction in hospital stay.

Pulmonary complications

Postoperatively, most patients show a major reduction in pulmonary function with lung volumes and flows depressed by 20–60 per cent of preoperative values. This is most obvious in patients who have undergone thoracic and upper-abdominal surgery. Coughing and clearing of secretions is markedly impaired when surgery is close to the diaphragm. In addition, since movement results in pain, the diaphragm is held taught and 'splinted'. Gas exchange is abnormal and the development of atelectasis and pneumonia result in significant morbidity.

Early studies looked only at intraoperative anaesthetic techniques—comparing epidural and general anaesthesia—and found no benefit in improved postoperative course. However, the use of continuous epidural local anaesthesia to provide postoperative pain relief showed improvements in pulmonary function and a reduction in pulmonary complications. These techniques have been shown to be better than conventional intramuscular morphine after abdominal and thoracic procedures. Opioid administration into the epidural space (see Chapter 11) instead of local anaesthetic solutions also appears to reduce pulmonary complications. Alternative local anaesthetic techniques such as intercostal nerve blockade or wound infiltration also produce improvements in postoperative pulmonary function.

Respiratory depression resulting from conventional opioid regimens may be a contributing factor to the development of pulmonary complications after surgery. However, it is clear that an aggressive approach to postoperative pain control can result in measurable improvements in pulmonary function and a reduction in complications. These effects are especially noticeable in high-risk groups such as patients who have had thoracic and upper-abdominal operations.

Stress response to surgery and trauma

There are characteristic endocrine and metabolic changes which occur after surgery, trauma, and infection. These responses have developed from the 'fear, fight, and flight' mechanisms developed to enable the body to survive following injury. The characteristic changes are listed in Table 3.1.

Table 3.1 Biochemical and endocrinological changes associated with the stress response to trauma and surgery

Increased pituitary hormone secretion	Increased	β endorphin ACTH GH Prolactin ADH
Sympathetic nervous system activation	Increased	Adrenalin Noradrenalin
Fluid and electrolyte changes		Sodium and water retention Elevated blood glucose
Skeletal muscle breakdown		Amino acids used in gluconeo-genesis and in the synthesis of acute-phase proteins

In general, increased catabolism is seen with the development of negative nitrogen balance associated with skeletal muscle breakdown. Lipolysis occurs and the patient will exhibit hyperglycaemia and impaired glucose tolerance. Changes in fluid balance will also be seen as a result of sodium and water retention.

Pain is believed to be a major component in the initiation of the stress response. Variations of anaesthetic techniques and their modifying effects upon the stress response have been studied. Epidural regional anaesthetic techniques have been shown to significantly blunt the stress response following lower-abdominal and lower-extremity surgery. Systemic opioids are only useful when administered in very high doses. Combinations of regional anaesthetic agents and opioids administered into the epidural space may be beneficial in upper-abdominal and thoracic surgery but may have to be given continuously.

Thromboembolic complications

Virchow described the triad of vascular damage, venous stasis, and hypercoagulability, which underlies the development of venous thrombosis. Patients undergoing orthopaedic operations on the lower limb and lower-abdominal and pelvic surgery are at particular risk of developing this complication. Pain encourages immobility, resulting in venous stasis, and this increases the risk of deep venous thrombosis.

Epidural anaesthesia and continuous postoperative epidural analgesic techniques reduce this complication by both improving the blood flow through the lower limbs by sympathetic blockade and modifying the endocrine/metabolic stress response to surgery and thereby reducing the hypercoagulable state.

Return of gastrointestinal function

Pain impairs gastrointestinal function and in particular delays gastric emptying. The use of parenteral opioids has also been associated with a reduction in gastrointestinal motility. When regional analgesic techniques or intrathecal and epidural morphine are used, an earlier return to normal bowel function is seen. Return of normal function as early as possible is desirable to maintain adequate nutrition and to reduce hospital stay.

Mental state

Patients at increased risk of postoperative deterioration of mental function include the elderly, in whom return of mental function is particularly important for mobilization and return to their home environment.

There remains controversy about the influence of anaesthetic drugs and techniques and postoperative analgesia on mental changes. It has been suggested that regional analgesic techniques which reduce or avoid the need for opioid drugs would be of benefit.

Cardiovascular function

For the patient with heart disease, pain represents an unnecessary stress on the myocardium. Numerous studies of anaesthetic techniques in this group of patients have shown reductions in ischaemic episodes when epidural techniques are combined with light general anaesthesia. Attention to postoperative analgesia by all methods can be expected to reduce morbidity and mortality by reducing sympathetic drive and catecholamine release.

Thoracic epidural techniques when used to provide postoperative analgesia improve myocardial function as a result of sympathetic blockade. This results in reductions in both pre-load and after-load and, in addition, coronary vessels dilate. This technique has also been reported to be of value in patients with crescendo angina that is uncontrolled by other pharmacological means. Improvement is seen not only in pain control but also in myocardial function.

4 Psychological aspects of acute pain

Pain is a subjective experience which has complex interactions with the emotional state of the patient. The concept of the pain experience as a whole can be considered at three distinct levels.

1. The first level is the sensory and discriminative input from the noxious stimulus via the sensory nervous system—the result of sticking your finger with a needle, for example.
2. At the second level motivational factors and the affective state of the patient (awake, asleep, happy, sad) can alter the interpretation of input at the central nervous system.
3. Thirdly, the evaluation of the stimulus by our thoughts or cognitions processes the overall response to the pain.

Approaches to the management of pain can therefore be seen as not only directed towards the sensory input but also to the emotional and other factors which influence the patient's response. This was described in early work by Beecher in 1956 (*a,b*) and has more recently been developed extensively in pain clinics, in the control of chronic pain.

A trimodal system of pain management has been described where the appropriate therapies available for pain control have been classified into three levels of intervention.

1. Cognitive strategies

- Imagery
- Attention diversion.

Cognitive strategies refer to techniques that influence the pain experience through the medium of thoughts or cognitions. These can be taught preoperatively to patients in preparation for surgery. They have been assessed using experimental pain techniques in volunteers where the studies can be performed before and after the teaching of cognitive controls. In this setting these techniques prolong the ability to withstand previously painful levels of experimental pain. Examples which have been used in these techniques include the following:

Distraction —imaging pleasant events
—focusing on other things
—concentrating on sensations other than pain.

Dissociation—dissociating from the pain (self hypnosis)
—imagining the affected area as numb.

Perhaps the most common use of psychological strategies to combat pain is in the preparation for childbirth. Behavioural and cognitive techniques are taught to pregnant women to reduce the effects of labour pain. Studies have shown that these techniques provide benefit particularly in the early stage of labour, although few women can still use these techniques by the time the second stage of labour is reached.

2. *Behavioural manipulations*

With behavioural strategies, patients exercise a response to the pain, giving them a feeling of control. This element of patient control was first described when nitrous oxide and air mixtures were used to diminish the pain of childbirth. This method recognized the importance of allowing patients to control their own analgesia. More recently the introduction of patient-controlled analgesia systems for use with opioid analgesics has highlighted the importance of this.

Other behavioural techniques which have been described may be useful in both acute and chronic pain. These can be divided into two types. A first group, which requires the presence of external people or features to derive best effects, includes the following.

● Hypnosis.

● Operant-conditioning techniques to reinforce helpful pain behaviours.

● Biofeedback training may be useful for recurrent pain problems such as Raynaud's phenomenon and migraine. It requires training of patients to enable them to change specific physiological parameters such as skin temperature and muscle tension.

● Modelling techniques: children can be helped by video tapes showing other children's appropriate responses to painful or unpleasant procedures.

A second group, which depends less on external controls, includes the following.

- Placebos: approximately 35 per cent of patients with acute pain will show a response to placebos.

- Perceived controllability: patients who have learnt to feel in control of pain themselves will respond better and report lower pain scores. Those who rely on external control will report higher pain scores.

3. Physical intervention

This describes the final level of methods available to influence pain and includes physical and pharmacological methods.

- Relaxation.

- Physiotherapy: this can include the applications of heat and cold by a variety of means, which may alleviate pain and reduce any associated muscle spasm.

- Transcutaneous nerve stimulation (p. 131).

- Acupuncture (p. 132).

- Pharmacological agents, opioids, non steroidal anti-inflammatory drugs, and local anaesthetics and inhalational agents (Chapters 6–15).

Patient features influencing pain control

Emotional and personality effects modify our response to pain at the brain level; they do not affect peripheral pain thresholds. The most commonly studied personality effects are extrovertism and neuroticism. Extroverts are generally believed to complain more about their pain and may be expected to receive more analgesics in clinical situations. Patients with high neurotic-scale scores may be seen to rate their pain much higher in studies.

Pain is not only associated with the idea of bodily harm but also more complex feelings of guilt, loss, and punishment that may be associated with the injury. A patient's strategy for responding to these conflicts may serve to worsen or alleviate the distress. The processes of denial, dissociation, and distraction may help alleviate pain whereas patients who catastrophize, characterized by negative attitudes and overly negative thoughts and ideas, will cope less well with their pain. These individual strategies will have been learnt from the patient's previous experience of pain and their socio-cultural development.

Knowledge and fears relating to the aetiology, pathology, treatment, and prognosis of their illness, misunderstandings, and inadequate information can lead to increased anxiety in patients. Their distress may not be obvious—remember 'the stiff-upper-lip attitude'. Recognition and clarification of these problems can reduce the emotional distress.

Anxiety

The influence of anxiety on pain perception and analgesic requirements has also been widely studied. Anxiety has been considered as arising from two sources.

State anxiety is that which arises from a particular stress and may be anticipatory or situational.

Trait anxiety is the tendency of an individual to respond to stress with high or low levels of anxiety. This will be modified by an individual's socio-cultural background, early experiences, prior conditioning, and developmental state. High levels of trait anxiety are associated with increased pain perception. A depressive affect may also influence postoperative pain. These effects may be seen even with minor levels of depression, which might be assumed as a normal variation.

Often obvious differences are seen in the degree and nature of anxiety that patients exhibit. Some will need frequent reassurance, and approach all members of staff; others may show unnatural stoicism or a feeling of virtue from suffering.

Patients preparing for surgery often have profound fears about anaesthesia, including the fear of losing control and ultimately of death, and these may be more important than the implications of the operation. Encouragement must be given to broach these fears however irrational they appear. Any previous traumatic anaesthetic or surgical experience must be appreciated so that anxiety may be allayed with sympathetic counselling.

Type of surgery

The type of surgery that the patient is about to undergo is a particularly important component of preoperative stress. Since the heart is still seen as the physical and emotional centre of life, cardiac surgery is seen as particularly threatening to the patient. Mutilating operations such as amputations and mastectomy and also some plastic surgery procedures which change body shape are more traumatic psychologically. The well-recognized 'fear of cancer' may be present in many patients before surgery. This may often be an irrational fear when the patient's symptoms and disease are incompatible with the diagnosis of cancer, and this anxiety may be relieved by careful explanation and reassurance. However, in some cases it may be impossible to reassure the patient, even if the prognosis of the type of neoplasia is good, until the histological diagnosis is received.

Preoperative discussion with the patient about the effects of their operation and the nature of the pain and other sensations that they will experience following recovery should include the methods available to alleviate pain. It may be too late, at this stage, for instruction in any psychological strategies to be effective.

Information must be presented in understandable form for each patient. Booklets and videos have been used to prepare patients for hospitalization and surgery but the patient's hospital attendants must be prepared to reinforce the information. Many patients will need support and information from all members of staff. The support of relatives also becomes an important source of information and reassurance to the patient.

Paediatrics

The young child may have complicated interpretations of illness depending on age and developmental level. Pain control in children has often suffered from the myths that young children do not feel pain or, if they do feel pain, do not remember it.

Several factors are important when assessing pain in children:

- developmental level;
- parental attitudes;
- effects of hospitalization;
- symbolic meaning of pain;
- physiological response to pain.

The developmental level of a child may limit his ability to communicate that he is in pain. Furthermore, the strange hospital environment and the child's shyness of strangers may inhibit him from asking for pain relief. Young children may perceive injections as assaults and be unable to appreciate that they are responsible for relieving the pain. Doctors and nurses may overestimate a child's understanding and the effects of illness and hospitalization may also produce regression to earlier developmental levels. Young children have a special concern about body integrity and fears of possible mutilation. In young children pain may be interpreted as a punishment. Special attention needs to be paid to children's fears when they are prepared for surgery. They can often be helped to adjust to hospital stays by careful preparation. Successful techniques which have been used to achieve this include video or social modelling, behaviour therapies, and hypnosis.

There has been considerable progress over the last 20 years in caring for children in hospital and an increased awareness of their particular problems. Parents are now able to stay with their children and participate in their care. Day-stay surgery, allowing children to spend shorter periods in hospital, has become increasingly popular and the environment of children's wards has become less threatening.

5 Principles of analgesic drug administration

This section briefly introduces important pharmacological terms which apply to the following chapters on analgesic drug use and administration.

Agonist

This term applies to an agent, which when combined with a receptor, produces a biological action.

Antagonist

This term is used for agents which will block the actions of agonist drugs.

Actions of both types of agent are often also described as competitive (or reversible) or non-competitive (irreversible) in their actions.

Agonist—antagonist agents

Opioid drugs of this type have agonist actions at one opioid receptor site and antagonist properties at another. Thus they can also be used as antagonists of pure agonist agents. Some of these agents, as a result of their antagonist properties, can produce symptoms of opioid withdrawal syndromes in dependent patients.

Bioavailability

This term applies to the percentage of an oral dose which reaches the systemic circulation. It depends upon the extent of drug absorption and the amount of drug undergoing metabolism on first pass through the gut wall or the liver. The term can also be applied to doses given by other routes such as rectal or buccal administration.

Clearance

This expression denotes the volume of plasma cleared of drug per unit time. It is a composite of both hepatic metabolism and renal excretion and elimination by other organs.

Dependence

Fear of addiction

This is often expressed as a concern by people involved in the prescribing and administering of opioids in acute pain. It is an irrational fear and is an important cause of inadequate analgesia being administered to patients in pain. The Boston Collaborative Drug Surveillance programme reviewed the records of 11 882 hospital patients who had received at least one narcotic preparation. Results showed only four reasonably well-documented cases of addiction in patients with no previous history of drug abuse—an incidence of 0.03 per cent.

When opioid drugs are administered for prolonged periods for chronic pain problems they are often restricted to terminal care patients. Even in this situation the incidence of addiction to the drugs is low and, when it has occurred, has been easily managed.

Physical dependence

This phenomenon is demonstrated by the appearance of symptoms and signs of withdrawal (or abstinence) syndrome if the drug is abruptly discontinued or opioid antagonists are administered to patients after prolonged opioid use. These effects include sweating, tachycardia, and diarrhoea. The severity of the withdrawal effects is dependent upon the dose and duration of previous opioid administration.

Psychic dependence

This term is used to describe the compulsive drug-seeking behaviour exhibited with addiction. This occurs with opioids primarily as a result of their mood-altering effects. However, drug use for medical purposes is not a major factor in the development of addiction. When opioids are used to relieve acute pain the development of addiction is rare. Other medical, social, psychological, economic, and cultural factors play important roles in addiction.

First-pass metabolism

Some drugs when given orally may undergo significant metabolism on first pass through the gut wall, liver, or both. This can be a variable amount in some patients and may be influenced by hepatic blood flow and disease states. There may be up to five-fold increases in plasma drug concentrations in patients with cirrhosis who have porto-systemic shunting due to a reduction in hepatic metabolism. The effect of first-pass metabolism means that to produce equivalent effects, an oral dose will need to be considerably greater than a parenteral dose.

Half life

This is defined as the time taken for the plasma concentration of a drug to decrease by half. After intravenous doses a typical plot of plasma concentration against time would be as shown by Fig. 5.1. From such a graph the half lives of both the initial rapid distribution phase and of the slower elimination phase can be determined.

Opiate/opioid

The term opiate was originally applied to drugs obtained from the opium compound. These include morphine, codeine, and the semi-synthetic congeners of morphine. Following the development of totally synthetic drugs with morphine-like actions the term opioid was developed. It now stands as the generic designation for all exogenous substances that bind to any of the several sub-types of opioid receptors and produce agonist actions. However, in many texts the terms opioid and opiate are used interchangeably.

Partial agonists

These agents have agonist properties at low doses which do not increase with higher dosages. They have a low intrinsic efficacy

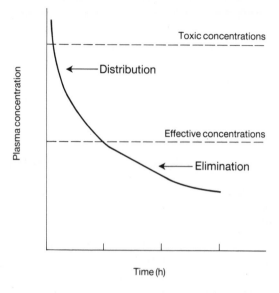

Fig. 5.1   Graph of plasma concentration plotted against time after intravenous
bolus of analgesic

and so opioid partial agonists, such as buprenorphine, exhibit a
ceiling effect to their analgesic effects.

Potency

The response to a drug is usually plotted on a dose-response
curve. A variety of drugs with the same actions can be compared
using these graphs. The most potent drug will produce its pharmacological effects at lower doses. However, the low potency of an
individual drug can be overcome by increasing the dosages used.

Tolerance

The development of tolerance is seen after a drug has been administered for some time and a given dose of drug produces a
decreasing effect. Thus larger doses of the drug are required to
produce the original level of effect. With opioid analgesics the
first indication of tolerance may be a reduction in the duration of

effect. As tolerance to analgesia develops so too does tolerance to the sedative and respiratory depressant effects of opioids. However, tolerance to the smooth-muscle effects of opioids, for example constipation, is slow to develop. Fortunately, with acute pain, in the majority of patients, pain will be decreasing over the time that tolerance develops.

Pharmacological factors important in analgesic drug administration

Changes in the effects of drugs may be the result of changes in the concentration of free drug available at the site of action resulting from altered pharmacokinetics (the effect of the body on drugs). Alternatively individual sensitivity to drugs may result from alterations at the receptor level where the drug acts (pharmacodynamics). Disease states may also predispose to altered sensitivity which may be through alterations in receptor sensitivity.

Age also affects many of the variables mentioned above resulting in increased sensitivity to many drugs in the elderly patient. With analgesic drugs, hepatic metabolism and renal excretion may be reduced and also altered receptor sensitivity may be responsible for reduced drug requirements. Neonates and infants under six months have increased sensitivity to the depressant effects of opioids. Reduced hepatic metabolism and increased permeability of the blood–brain barrier to drugs may be responsible.

When an analgesic drug has been administered the amount of drug remaining in the body at any given time will depend on the following factors:

- route of administration;
- frequency of administration;
- rate of release of the drug from its formulation;
- rate of absorption from the site of administration;
- the amount of metabolism that occurs in the gut wall or liver as the drug is absorbed (first-pass metabolism);
- the rate of distribution to organs and tissues;
- routes and rates of metabolism;
- routes and rates of excretion.

As well as inter-individual differences in these factors in any individual patient disease states may also alter any of the above variables.

ROUTES OF ADMINISTRATION OF ANALGESIC DRUGS

In clinical practice several routes are available for analgesic administration. These are discussed in this chapter.

Parenteral routes of drug administration

Intravenous injection

The intravenous route is the most important route for analgesic drug administration in the treatment of acute pain. Its advantages include the immediate access of the drug to the circulation, ensuring complete availability and rapid onset of action. It may be used for single intravenous doses (bolus) or for the administration of drugs by continuous infusion.

There are disadvantages with this route, which include

- the need to secure intravenous access and the maintenance of this access for prolonged periods;
- the need for medical staff or specially trained nurses to be available to administer intravenous boluses;
- the possibility that the drug may be more rapidly eliminated, thereby shortening its duration of action.

Intramuscular injection

This is the commonest parenteral route used for the administration of opioid analgesic drugs on hospital wards. The standard prescription for analgesia is usually for intramuscular injections of an opioid analgesic given four-hourly as required. This has many disadvantages. The patient must express a demand for analgesia. Few patients can anticipate the end of the analgesic effect of the drugs and will therefore be in pain before each demand is met. In addition a standard time of four hours between doses may be too long for healthy, young adults but be too short a time interval for elderly patients. It has gained acceptance because it does not require medical supervision for its administration and is simple to give.

When administered by this route the rate of absorption of the drugs is dependent upon muscle blood flow. The onset of effects will therefore be slower than after intravenous injection. Additional disadvantages include the pain caused by the injections and the risks of major bruising in patients with a bleeding diathesis. Injections at inappropriate sites in the buttocks and thigh have been known to result in vascular and neural damage.

Subcutaneous injection

The subcutaneous route provides an accessible parenteral route for the administration of analgesic drugs. The absorption of drug from the subcutaneous site is dependent upon regional skin blood flow and this may make it unsuitable for use in patients where skin perfusion is reduced, particularly the shocked, hypovolaemic patient. More recently the use of small cannulae placed subcutaneously has allowed this route to be used for repeated intermittent dosing or for continuous infusion of drugs.

Drugs administered subcutaneously may be irritant and the injection can be painful. In some cases pyogenic abscess formation may occur.

Oral

This is the standard route of administration for most drugs. However, this route is often not practicable when treating acute pain. Pain itself reduces gastric emptying, making this route ineffective. Postoperative vomiting and gastrointestinal stasis will also render the oral route unsuitable. In the unco-operative or unconscious patients the oral route will not be available although some patients may have a nasogastric tube in place which may be used.

The need to achieve analgesia rapidly in the distressed patient is of considerable importance. Drugs given by the oral route are dependent upon the physical dissolution of the drug formulation, the rate of gastric emptying, and gastrointestinal motility before absorption takes place through the mucosa of the small intestine. The rate of gastric emptying and gastrointestinal motility may be delayed postoperatively or as a result of opioid administration, therefore limiting its use. However, the use of an oral slow-release preparation of analgesic, perhaps administered preoperatively, may be helpful in providing analgesia in the early postoperative period. Suitable drugs include slow-release morphine or some non-steroidal anti-inflammatory analgesics. The opioid drugs, in particular, are subject to extensive first-pass metabolism when given by the oral route and the doses required to produce equivalent analgesia are considerably greater than by parenteral routes. Three to six times the dose of morphine may be required to be given orally as compared with the intramuscular route to produce equivalent effects.

Commonly, acute pain gradually improves over a period of 2–3 days. Initially patients may require parenteral therapy with opioid analgesics, but as requirements for analgesia reduce, the patient may be managed with oral opioids, non-steroidal anti-inflammatory drugs, or combinations of these drugs, providing gastrointestinal absorption is adequate.

Non-parenteral routes of drug administration

To overcome the inability to use the oral route to provide analgesia, alternative non-parenteral routes of administration including sublingual, buccal, rectal, transdermal, and intranasal may be utilized.

Sublingual/buccal

The advantages of these routes of administration include avoiding first-pass metabolism of drugs, avoiding the need for injections whilst remaining independent of effects on gastric emptying, vomiting, and gastrointestinal motility. They are acceptable to patients because they avoid the pain of injections, although some co-operation is required in preventing chewing or swallowing of the drug preparation. Drugs can be formulated as a tablet, solution, or paste, which influence their rate of absorption through the oral mucous membranes. Absorption through the buccal mucosa of some opioids is rapid and because first-pass metabolism is avoided, most of the drug is available for analgesia.

Taste is obviously important in patient acceptance of these routes of administration, many of the opioids producing a bitter taste when given sublingually or buccally, thus limiting their use. Problems may occur with both of these routes in patients with reduced saliva production, which makes dissolution of tablet preparations slow. Some drug will be lost by chewing and swallowing even with good patient co-operation. If there is delayed gastric emptying, this may produce a considerable depot of analgesic drug in the stomach, which may be rapidly absorbed once gastrointestinal function is restored.

Rectal

This is a further route which utilizes the end portion of the gastrointestinal tract without the disadvantages of oral administration. The use of the rectal route has not gained wide patient acceptance in British medical practice although it enjoys great popularity in other countries. Slow absorption of the drug preparation leads to a slow onset of analgesia—a disadvantage in the initial management of acute pain. Although first-pass metabolism is reduced the amount of drug that is available for analgesic purposes is variable.

The rectal route is well suited to the maintenance of analgesia and slow-release preparations are often used. It has gained popularity principally in providing analgesia in patients with chronic pain resulting from malignancy.

Transdermal

This is a new technique and few analgesic drugs are available at present. Topical application of non-steroidal anti-inflammatory drugs is being developed for local use in arthritic pain. An experimental delivery system for the synthetic opioid fentanyl has been developed, at which the rate limit is that of the release of the drug from the preparation providing a controlled-release infusion. Although still undergoing investigation, this route may prove useful for background analgesia to which small intermittent intravenous bolus doses may be added as necessary for severe pain.

Intranasal

This is also a recent experimental approach to drug administration and has been used with the short-acting synthetic opioid sufentanil in premedication. The drug is rapidly and effectively absorbed from the nasal mucosa and avoids the distress of intramuscular injections.

Epidural and intrathecal

Following the discovery of the opioid receptors in the substantia gelatinosa of the spinal cord the direct application of opioid drugs to this area was investigated and has proved successful in producing analgesia. The use of the epidural and intrathecal routes of administration in analgesia have increased. The theory, applications, and complications of these routes of administration are discussed in Chapter 11. Local anaesthetic agents may also be administered by these routes to provide analgesia (see Chapter 14).

For a comparison of the various drug administration routes available see Table 5.1.

Table 5.1   Advantages and disadvantages of the various routes available for analgesic drug administration

Route	Advantages	Disadvantages
Oral	No injections needed Can be used to give drugs preoperatively, e.g. slow-release opioids or NSAIDs	Fasting patients not suitable Nausea and vomiting reduces availability of this route Unpredictable absorption and bioavailability of drugs Reduced GI motility postoperatively Requires conscious and co-operative patient or nasogastric tube
Intravenous	Rapid onset Predictable effects Complete availability Suitable for continuous infusion techniques	Intravenous access is required Qualified nursing staff or medical staff required to give drugs High peak-plasma concentrations may be associated with increased side effects and more rapid metabolism

Intramuscular	Standard route used in wards	Intermittent technique
		Painful injections
	No specialist staff required to administer drugs by this route	Risk of nerve/vascular damage
		Variable rate of absorption
	Relatively rapid onset of analgesia	
Subcutaneous	Relatively easy access—small cannulae can be used for repeat doses	Variable absorption particularly if reduced skin blood flow, shock, etc.
	Route may be used for continuous infusions	Irritant and painful injections
		Abscess formation is a risk
		Depot remaining in skin after infusions discontinued
Sublingual/buccal	Bypass first-pass elimination	Patient co-operation not to chew or swallow the preparation
	Independent of gastric emptying or nausea and vomiting	Dissolution of tablets slow if reduced saliva production
	High patient acceptability	Taste important for acceptance
Rectal	Reduced first-pass metabolism	Low patient acceptance
	Slow-release preparations useful	Slow absorption and slow onset of effect—not helpful for acute pain
	Independent of gastric emptying and nausea and vomiting	Bioavailability is variable and unpredictable
	Reduced risk of GI side effects with NSAIDs	
Transdermal	Slow release—useful for background analgesia	New route—few drugs available

	Variable formulations to produce different rates of drug release	Absorption slow, onset of analgesia delayed
		Depot remains in skin when preparation removed
		Difficult to titrate against acute pain
Inhalational	Rapid onset and recovery	Prolonged use associated with bone marrow depression
	Moderately potent analgesic	Pollution of working environment
	Useful for intermittent administration and episodic pain of short duration	Patient co-operation required
		Patient variability—some will have excess sedation
Epidural/spinal	see Chapters 11 and 14	

6   Opioid pharmacology

Opioid agents have effects on many systems in the body. This chapter describes some of these effects.

CENTRAL NERVOUS SYSTEM EFFECTS

Opioid agents have a variety of effects on the central nervous system, which can be broadly classified as depressant or excitatory effects.

Depressant effects

Analgesia

This is the most common indication for the therapeutic use of opioid drugs. It results from the action of opiates at a number of levels in the central nervous system, listed below:

1. Direct effects at spinal cord level in the dorsal horn region.
2. They may influence the descending inhibitory pathways in the brain stem.
3. They are recognized to have mood-elevating effects acting through the limbic system.

Respiratory depression

This results from depression of the respiratory centres found in the medulla which have a reduced response to carbon dioxide. A slow respiratory pattern, with large tidal volumes, is characteristic of opioid-induced respiratory depression.

Sedation

Drowsiness is a common feature of opiate use. It may be due to the direct effect of opioids and also to the relief of pain and reduced perception of external stimuli. Occasionally euphoriant properties predominate, resulting from a paradoxical excitation usually due to depression of central inhibitory pathways.

Cough suppression

This was a previously widely used indication for opioid therapy and this action of opioids is still used in patients needing ventilatory support. Suppression of coughing results from the action of opioids on medullary cough centres. It is not a universal property of opioids but appears to be related to particular chemical configurations—codeine and diamorphine are more effective than morphine. The antitussive effects of the opioid drugs may be a useful adjunct to their analgesic effects in critically ill patients who require tracheal intubation.

Excitatory effects

Pupillary constriction

All opioids stimulate the Edinger–Westphal nucleus of the occulomotor nerve, resulting in miosis.

Nausea and vomiting

This may result from a combination of opioid drug effects. There is direct stimulation of the chemoreceptor trigger zone and the vomiting centre situated in the medulla and brain stem. These effects are potentiated by vestibular stimulation hence the worsening of nausea and vomiting once patients become more mobile.

CARDIOVASCULAR EFFECTS

In normal therapeutic doses the cardiovascular effects of opiate drugs are minimal. Bradycardia may be seen with morphine and fentanyl, whereas pethidine has weak atropine-like effects resulting in a slight increase in heart rate. Vasodilatation as a result of depression of the medullary vasomotor centres may occur. In addition, morphine has a direct vasodilatory effect on resistance and capacitance vessels.

GASTROINTESTINAL EFFECTS

Opioids cause contraction of smooth muscle throughout the gastrointestinal tract. Gastric emptying is delayed, intestinal transit time is prolonged, and there may be spasm of the anal sphincter.

A well recognized but infrequent problem is the occasional production of symptoms suggestive of biliary colic after opioid administration. These occur as a result of spasm of the biliary tree and sphincter of Oddi and an increase in intrabiliary pressure. Pethidine does not cause the same increase in intrabiliary pressure as does morphine, although its effects on biliary spasm are still significant. These properties have led to the use of pethidine as the first-line opioid analgesic for the pain of biliary colic.

URINARY TRACT EFFECTS

The detrusor muscle in the bladder and urinary sphincter at the exit of the bladder may contract in response to opioids, leading to urgency and inability to void. Urinary retention is more common in men. It is a frequent problem after the epidural administration of opioids.

HISTAMINE RELEASE

Allergic responses to opioids are extremely rare. Morphine, pethidine, and codeine are all known to release histamine, which may result in vasodilatation. The cutaneous manifestations of histamine release may also be seen; these include erythema, pruritis, urticaria, and bronchospasm.

Symptoms resulting from allergic reactions to opiates may include sweating, nausea, chest pain, and palpitations. Transient loss of consciousness may occur as a result of hypotension. In patients who demonstrate allergic reactions to opioids there may be some cross sensitivity between individual agents.

RESPIRATORY EFFECTS

The clinical significance of respiratory depression

This is the most significant unwanted effect of opioid drugs and remains a barrier to effective pain control. Warning signs are seen well in advance of the situation becoming dangerous. With careful monitoring of patients receiving opioids the problem can be minimized.

Investigation of opioid-induced respiratory depression has often been undertaken in healthy volunteers, patients undergoing anaesthesia, or preoperative patients. The influence of pain, anaesthetic drugs, and surgical interventions on respiratory function are important factors that are rarely considered in such studies. The interrelationship of these factors and opioid use are complex.

The respiratory-depressant effects of opioids vary, not only with different agents, but also with the same agent given by different routes of administration. The lower doses of opioids required to produce analgesia when administered by the spinal route may produce less respiratory depression than systemic administration. However, when these effects do occur after spinal administration they may be delayed.

The use of intravenous infusions of opioids may provide improved analgesia but when compared with standard intermittent intramuscular injections this technique is associated with increased episodes of slow respiratory rates and apnoea. Similarly, postoperative analgesic methods using opioids when compared with those using local-anaesthetic techniques result in increased episodes of arterial oxygen desaturation, indicating intermittent respiratory insufficiency. These episodes occur most commonly when patients are asleep, which appears to have an additive effect on opioid-induced respiratory depression. Supplemental oxygen will reduce the incidence of arterial desaturation but abnormalities of respiratory rate and apnoea will persist.

The standard monitoring of respiratory function on the ward usually consists of intermittent measures of respiratory rate by nursing staff. This will be inadequate to detect transient events or apnoeic episodes after opioid therapy. Furthermore some patients may have normal respiratory rates but still be hypoxic or hypercarbic. If other measurements such as pulse and blood pressure, which disturb the patient, are combined with respiratory rate measures, then true resting effects will not be monitored.

Direct tests for measuring respiratory effects can be time consuming, require patient co-operation, and their reliability as predictors of clinical deterioration is uncertain. Indirect measures are therefore the most widely used in clinical practice. Oximetry is the best indirect method available for monitoring arterial oxygen saturation (SaO_2). This equipment uses the differential absorption of light by saturated and desaturated haemoglobin to produce a continuous display of pulse and oxygen saturation. Sensors are comfortable for the patients and can be used for long-term monitoring. The equipment has a rapid response time to changing saturations. Normal saturation levels are of the order of 95–99 per cent (equivalent to a partial pressure of oxygen in arterial blood (PaO_2) of >10 kPa) and the equipment is accurate to low saturations of 70 per cent ($PaO_2 < 7$ kPa).

Transcutaneous measurements of PaO_2 and $PaCO_2$ have proved reliable in children and have been widely used in neonatal intensive care. Their use in adults is difficult, as variations in skin thickness influence the results. The sensors heat up the skin resulting in the need for frequent changes of site to reduce the risk of burns, particularly in the small premature infant.

In patients who are at high risk of developing respiratory complications, such as patients with chest injuries or following thoracic and upper-abdominal surgery in patients with pre-existing pulmonary disease, or in patients requiring ventilatory support, indwelling arterial cannula allows frequent sampling for arterial blood-gas analysis. It is the most reliable method of assessment of respiratory function especially when combined with continuous SaO_2 monitoring. Without this facility the use of continuous or intermittent SaO_2 monitoring is the best alternative.

7 Useful opioid analgesic drugs

The analgesic and euphoric properties of opium have been known for several thousand years. The word 'opium' is derived from the Greek, meaning juice. The source of the juice being the unripe seed-heads of the poppy *Papaver somniferum*. Despite the years of use and abuse its derivatives still remain in the forefront of our armamentarium today for the treatment of pain.

Properties of an ideal opioid

The ideal agent for analgesic use should have

- rapid onset of analgesic effect;
- no accumulation following prolonged administration;
- safe and reliable elimination even with impaired hepatic or renal function;
- lack of acute or chronic toxicity, enzyme induction, or tachyphylaxis;
- no depression of respiration;
- cardiovascular stability;
- no adverse endocrinological effects;
- no increase in muscle tone;
- no venous irritation;
- high therapeutic ratio;
- lack of active metabolites;
- simple administration by all routes IM/IV/subcutaneous/oral;
- no addictive potential;
- no absorption on to plastic or glass;
- no interactions with other drugs;
- water soluble—so that effects of solvents can be ignored;
- stable in solution and on exposure to light, allowing easy storage;
- low cost;

- the same bioavailability when given by all routes so that drug dosage does not depend on route of administration.

Currently used drugs

Table 7.1 lists the dosage equivalents of opioids discussed in this and the subsequent chapter.

Table 7.1 Dosage equivalents for opioids in cases of severe pain

Opioid	Equianalgesic dose	Dose interval
Fentanyl	100 μg IV	0.5-1 h
Morphine	10 mg IM	3-4 h
Papaveretum	20 mg IM	3-4 h
Diamorphine	5 mg IM	3-4 h
Pethidine	100 mg IM	3-4 h
Buprenorphine	0.3-0.6 mg IM	6-8 h
Methadone	10 mg IM	8-12 h

Morphine

Morphine was originally identified by Serturner, a German chemist, in 1805. It is the standard agent against which the activity of all other analgesics may be measured and remains the most valuable opioid analgesic. Its chemical structure is shown in Fig. 7.1. Early attempts at modification of the morphine molecule led to the synthesis of diamorphine and hydromorphone and the discovery of codeine.

In the treatment of acute, severe pain, morphine may be given intravenously or intramuscularly. The standard dose is 10 mg/70 kg repeated four-hourly intramuscularly. When given intravenously, smaller doses of 2–5 mg should be given and repeated after 5–10 min until adequate analgesia has been obtained. Opioid drugs are generally not recommended for infants under six months, unless they are in an intensive-care environment, as this group appear to be extremely sensitive to the respiratory-depressant effects. The recommended dose of morphine for older children is 0.15–0.2 mg/kg.

Oral preparations of morphine are available; however, morphine undergoes significant first-pass metabolism. When morphine is

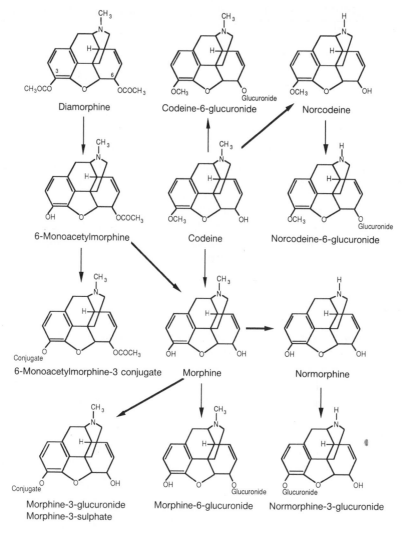

Fig. 7.1 Chemical structures of morphine, diamorphine, and codeine, and their metabolites

given orally, 20–30 mg is equivalent to 10 mg given by the intramuscular route. New oral preparations of morphine (Sevredol, Napp Laboratories Ltd) may prove useful in the management of acute pain.

The duration of effective analgesia obtained from morphine is approximately three hours.

Adult doses:	2–5 mg IV
	5–10 mg IM
	30–40 mg oral.
Paediatrics:	0.02 mg/kg IV
	0.2 mg/kg IM.
Onset of action:	15–20 min IM
	5–10 min IV.
Duration of action:	3 h.

Morphine is metabolized principally in the liver to morphine 3-glucuronide and morphine 6-glucuronide. A small proportion is excreted unchanged via the kidney. The metabolite morphine 6-glucuronide is also pharmacologically active and may accumulate in patients with renal failure.

Papaveretum

This agent is often prescribed perioperatively for analgesia and is widely used as a premedicant drug for many types of operation. It is a mixture of alkaloids of opium and contains 47.5–52.5 per cent anhydrous morphine, anhydrous codeine 2.5–5.0 per cent, noscapine 16–22 per cent, and papaverine 2.5–7.0 per cent.

It is usually administered intramuscularly but may also be given intravenously.

20 mg of papaveretum is equivalent to 12.5 mg of morphine.

Adult doses:	2–5 mg IV
	10–20 mg IM.
Paediatrics:	0.04 mg/kg IV
	0.4 mg/kg IM.
Onset of action:	15–20 min IM
	5–10 min IV.
Duration of action:	3 h.

Diamorphine

The chemical structure of diamorphine is shown in Fig. 7.1. It differs from the structure of morphine in that the two hydroxyl groups in positions 3 and 6 are replaced by acetyl groups. These increase the lipid solubility of diamorphine, which allows it to penetrate rapidly into brain tissue. Once administered the diamorphine is rapidly de-acetylated to produce 6-monoacetyl morphine, which rapidly diffuses into the brain, and then finally to morphine. These metabolites are responsible for the analgesic effects of diamorphine.

Diamorphine is available in both oral and parenteral preparations. Its high degree of solubility, allowing high concentrations to be available in small volumes, is an asset.

When given by intramuscular injection, peak plasma concentrations are obtained within 10 min. After intravenous administration the drug is rapidly distributed producing a more rapid onset of action in comparison to morphine. It is also said to produce less nausea and vomiting than morphine and is more often associated with pleasant psychic effects. It is used parenterally for the treatment of acute pain of many forms and has been used to provide analgesia following acute myocardial infarction.

5 mg of diamorphine is equivalent to 10 mg of morphine.

Adult doses:	2-5 mg IM or IV.
Paediatrics:	0.1 mg/kg IM.
Onset of action:	5-10 min IM 2-5 min IV.
Duration of action:	3 h.

Methadone

This is a synthetic opioid with a prolonged duration of action and slow elimination. It undergoes little first-pass metabolism when administered by the oral route. The duration of analgesia is of the order of 6-8 h. However, accumulation will occur with frequent doses due to its prolonged elimination half life.

10 mg of methadone IM is equivalent to 10 mg of morphine. Oral doses of 10-15 mg are equianalgesic with oral doses of morphine in the range of 40-60 mg.

Adult doses:	5-10 mg IM.
Paediatrics:	Methadone is not recommended for use in children.

Onset of action: 10–15 min IM
                        30–60 min oral.

Duration of action: 6–8 h.

Pethidine

This drug is a synthetic opioid agonist which is a phenylpiperidine derivative. It undergoes rapid metabolism in the liver by microsomal oxidation and is therefore subject to extensive first-pass metabolism when given orally. One of its metabolites, norpethidine, is a central nervous system stimulant and may accumulate in patients with impaired renal function or in patients receiving prolonged infusions of pethidine, resulting in convulsions.

In comparison to other opioids, pethidine does not produce bradycardia by virtue of atropine-like effects at cholinergic nerve endings.

Drug interaction: If pethidine is given to patients receiving monoamine oxidase inhibitors, central nervous system excitation and hypertension or hypotension may occur.

100 mg of pethidine is equivalent to 10 mg of morphine.

Adult doses: 50–100 mg IM or IV
                        50–300 mg oral.

Paediatrics: 1 mg/kg IV
                        1.5–2 mg/kg IM.

Onset of action: 10–15 min IM
                        15–30 min oral.

Duration of action: 2 h.

Phenoperidine

This drug is a synthetic opioid agonist that is chemically related to pethidine. It is most frequently used as an adjunct to anaesthesia or in intensive care units for its analgesic and respiratory depressant effects in patients requiring mechanical ventilation. Unwanted central nervous system effects may be seen in patients with renal failure when phenoperidine may be metabolized to pethidine and subsequently to norpethidine, which will accumulate.

Phenoperidine 2 mg is equivalent to 10 mg of morphine.

Adult doses: 0.5–1 mg IV.

Paediatrics: 30–50 µg/kg.

In patients receiving assisted ventilation, doses of 1–2 mg (adults) or 100–150 µg/kg (children) may be repeated.

Onset of action: 2 min IV.

Duration of action: 40–60 min.

Fentanyl and derivatives

These drugs are newer synthetic opioid agonists that are chemically related to pethidine. In general they are drugs with a short duration of action. They are most commonly used during anaesthesia and for critically ill patients requiring intensive care. Due to their potency they should only be prescribed by the medical staff working in these disciplines.

Fentanyl There is little cardiovascular depression with this drug although a vagally mediated slowing of heart rate may occasionally be seen. It may also be administered into the epidural space to provide analgesia (see Chapter 11).

100 µg of fentanyl is equivalent to 10 mg of morphine.

Adult doses: 50–200 µg IV.

Paediatrics: 1–3 µg/kg IV.

Higher doses may be required in critically ill patients receiving assisted ventilation.

Onset of action: 1–2 min IV.

Duration of action: 30–60 min.

Alfentanil Alfentanil has a rapid onset of action with a very short duration of effect. It is often used as a perioperative analgesic agent for patients undergoing outpatient surgical procedures, because of its short action and rapid rate of metabolism. Its rapid metabolism has led to it being used in infusion systems, providing analgesia with low risk of drug accumulation.

1 mg of alfentanil is equivalent to 10 mg of morphine.

Adult doses:	up to 500 μg IV.
Paediatrics:	30–50 μg/kg IV.
Onset of action:	1–2 min IV.
Duration of action:	15–20 min.

Codeine

This drug is unusual as an opioid agonist in that it still retains high oral efficacy due to low first-pass metabolism. Approximately 10 per cent of the dose is metabolized to morphine and this may be the source of its analgesic properties. The remainder of the dose is metabolized to codeine-6-glucuronide. Codeine itself has a low affinity for the μ receptors.

120 mg of codeine IM is equianalgesic to 10 mg morphine.

Adult doses:	30–60 mg IM 30–60 mg oral.
Paediatrics:	3 mg/kg IM daily in divided doses.
Onset of action:	30–60 min orally 10–15 min IM.
Duration of action:	4–6 h.

Dihydrocodeine This agent is of similar structure and potency to codeine and may be given orally or intramuscularly.

60 mg is equivalent to 10 mg morphine IM.

Adult doses:	50 mg IM 30 mg oral.
Paediatrics:	0.5–1 mg/kg.
Onset of action:	30–60 min orally 15–20 min IM.
Duration of action:	4–5 h.

As a result of their oral efficacy, codeine and dihydrocodeine are often used in the management of moderate pain when parenteral administration is unnecessary.

PARTIAL AGONIST DRUGS

Buprenorphine

This drug is a semi-synthetic derivative of thebaine, an alkaloid of opium. It is a partial agonist at the μ receptor. Although it has a high affinity for the μ receptor it has a low intrinsic efficacy. It is rapidly absorbed after intramuscular injection or sublingual administration and peak plasma concentrations are found within five minutes of the intramuscular dose.

Respiratory depression may be seen with buprenorphine. This is not readily reversed by naloxone (the specific opioid antagonist) and the use of a non-specific respiratory stimulant such as doxapram, or ventilatory support, may be required. Side effects including sweating, nausea and vomiting, and dizziness can be troublesome.

0.4 mg IM is equianalgesic with 10 mg morphine.

Adult doses:	0.4–0.8 mg sublingually 0.3–0.6 mg IM.
Onset of action:	5 min IM/sublingual.
Duration of action:	6–8 h.

AGONIST/ANTAGONIST DRUGS

Pentazocine

This drug is a synthetic opioid with a benzomorphan structure, and is a weak μ antagonist and $\varkappa$ agonist. It exhibits a ceiling effect to its analgesic actions and also to its respiratory-depressant effects.

30 mg is equivalent to 10 mg IM morphine. 50 mg orally is equivalent to 60 mg of codeine.

Adult doses:	30–60 mg IM 25–50 mg oral.
Paediatrics:	1 mg/kg IM.

Onset of action: 15 min IM
                       1 h oral.

Duration of action: 3–4 h.

Nalbuphine

The analgesic effects of this agent result from its $\varkappa$-agonist activity. Structurally it is related to naloxone and oxymorphone. It exhibits marked antagonistic activity at μ receptors. The ceiling effect on respiratory depression is also seen. Dysphoria is less common unless high doses are used.

10 mg IM is equianalgesic with 10 mg morphine.

Adult doses: 10 mg IM/IV.

Paediatrics: 300 μg/kg IM/IV.

Onset of action: 10–15 min IM.

Duration of action: 3–4 h.

Meptazinol

This drug is also an agonist/antagonist combination and it is reputed to have a low incidence of respiratory depression in therapeutic doses. Nausea and vomiting are its principal adverse effects. Its use has been advocated in obstetrics as an alternative analgesic to pethidine for pain relief in labour.

100 mg IM is equianalgesic to 10 mg morphine.

Adult doses: 75–100 mg IM
                      200 mg oral.

Paediatrics: not recommended.

Onset of action: 15 min IM
                      1 h oral.

Duration of action: 3–4 h, with reports of up to 7 h.

Opioid antagonist drugs

Naloxone

This is the only agent in general use. It is a competitive antagonist at the μ, δ, κ, and σ receptors. Opioid antagonists will also block the analgesic response to placebo and also that obtained from the low-frequency acupuncture stimulation. It is thought that these effects are mediated through blockade of the endogenous opioid peptide systems. Naloxone also reverses the psychotomimetic and dysphoric effects of opioid drugs but higher doses are required (10–15 mg).

Small doses of naloxone (see below) will rapidly reverse respiratory depression. Sedation is reversed and an increase in respiratory rate may be observed within 1–2 min. Sudden reversal of analgesia is not without risk. Vomiting, emergence delirium, dysrhythmias, and pulmonary oedema have been reported in patients after surgery. These unwanted effects may result from a sudden outpouring of catecholamines such as adrenalin when analgesia is rapidly reversed. Naloxone will also precipitate an intense withdrawal state in patients who are physically dependent on opioids.

Management of respiratory depression

When given to patients who have opioid-induced respiratory depression, 0.4 mg of naloxone should be diluted in 10 ml of 0.9 per cent of saline and administered in divided doses. Doses of 1 ml should be given over a period of 15 s and repeated. Once the respiratory depression is reversed no further naloxone should be administered. Naloxone is metabolized in the liver and has a short duration of action—around 30 min–1 h.

Due to a short duration of action, repeated bolus doses of naloxone may be needed and these may be given intramuscularly or subcutaneously if necessary.

Naltrexone

This drug is an opioid antagonist which retains its activity following oral doses and has a prolonged duration of action. It is used only in the treated opioid addicts as an aid to maintaining their drug-free state.

8 Intramuscular administration of analgesics

The commonest, current practice, on most hospital wards, is to prescribe an analgesic drug on an 'as required' basis. Generally opioid analgesics are administered by the intramuscular route with a dosage interval varying from four to six hours. Many studies have reported the poor quality of analgesia provided by these standard regimes.

Intramuscular administration has gained acceptance because it is relatively simple to perform and does not require nurses with specialist training or medical staff. The *'as required'* prescription has achieved popularity for reasons which include the following.

- Fear of overdose—the staff have control over the number of doses administered.
- It is easy to give and requires fewer doses than regular administration.
- Administration occurs as a result of a patient demand and therefore the regime is often thought to be optimal.

As a result of widespread use and familiarity with the technique it is generally safe but often ineffective. Although the dose may be sufficient, given intermittently, on an 'as required' basis, by the intramuscular route there can be long periods when the patient will be in pain. This is a result of the lag time between demands for analgesia and the absorption and distribution of the drug after intramuscular injection producing effective analgesia. Even when prescribed four-hourly, most patients will receive only three doses in 24 h. Furthermore, this regimen can be inflexible, and standard doses may not be well suited to control pain of irregular severity. A rigid regime may not take account of inter-individual variations in analgesic requirements, or variations within the individual patient with time.

The analgesia provided by intermittent intramuscular injections could be improved by:

- more frequent administration;
- regular administration;
- depot preparations of opioids;
- opioids with long duration of action such as buprenorphine.

More frequent administration of analgesics, especially before painful procedures, or regular injections given before the pain has recurred, will benefit the patient. The time during which the patient is in pain will be reduced, and if observations of the patient's general condition and pain control are made before each administration (with appropriate guidelines for withholding doses), then overdosage is unlikely. It should be remembered that acute pain decreases with time and therefore prescriptions for regular opioid administration should have a limited time span (24–36 h) and be regularly reviewed.

Long-acting opioids may be useful in improving pain control when given intramuscularly. The partial agonist buprenorphine has a duration of analgesia of 6–8 h after intramuscular injection. It may also be prescribed to be given regularly at six-hourly intervals. Methadone also has a prolonged duration of action and this drug may accumulate, if given too frequently, and the interval between doses should be increased with regular administration.

Sites for intramuscular injections

The commonest sites for administration of intramuscular injections are the buttock and the thigh. In some patients the deltoid region may also be used. Complications of intramuscular injections include the following.

- Excessive bruising when patients have coagulation disturbances or are receiving anticoagulant therapy.
- When injections are made into the buttocks there is danger of damage to the sciatic nerve. This is the largest nerve in the body and enters the region of the buttock approximately midway between the ischial tuberosity and the greater trochanter

and then travels vertically down the back of the thigh to the popliteal fossa. The safe area for injections into the buttocks is the upper outer quadrant, remembering that the full extent of the buttock region includes the area upwards to the iliac crest and laterally to the greater trochanter.

In summary, present intramuscular opioid administration is generally safe and convenient but provides poor analgesia in some patients in acute pain. Recognition of its failings and improvements in technique may alleviate some of these problems. Regular assessment of the patient is essential to ensure adequate analgesia and maintain patient safety.

9 Opioid infusions

The standard prescription of intermittent analgesic drug regimens commonly leads to inadequate pain control. Improvement may be achieved using some form of continuous analgesic drug administration technique. This may have several advantages including

- avoidance of troughs in plasma drug concentrations (resulting in pain) which occur with intermittent dosage schedules;
- avoidance of high peak plasma concentrations (causing adverse effects) after bolus administration.

Continuous intravenous infusions should result in a constant level of analgesia for the duration of the infusion, avoiding periods of inadequate pain relief and periods of excessive sedation from intermittent high concentrations of drug by the administration of repeated bolus doses.

Pharmacokinetics of drug administration

When a continuous intravenous infusion is given, concentrations of drug in the plasma increase slowly with time. At a fixed rate of infusion it will take five times the elimination half life of the drug to reach 95 per cent of the steady-state plasma concentration.

A *low* rate of infusion may only reach an effective concentration once it has reached steady state.

A *high* rate of infusion will reach effective concentrations more quickly but will equilibrate at a toxic steady-state concentration.

To achieve therapeutic concentrations rapidly it is common to start the infusion at a high rate for a short period of time, then reduce it to one or two lower rates and then to a final maintenance rate. Alternatively, a loading dose of the drug can be given as a bolus and the infusion commenced at a maintenance rate (Fig. 9.1).

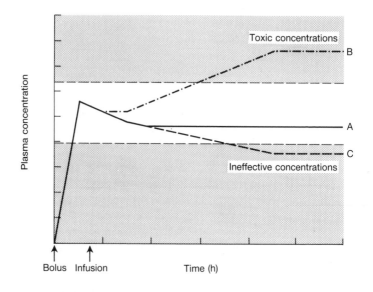

Fig. 9.1 Graph showing plasma concentration plotted against time after initial bolus, for continuous intravenous infusions after the same loading dose of analgesic. Plasma concentrations in the upper shaded area are toxic, those in the lower shaded area are ineffective. Thus curve A shows the ideal infusion rate; curve B shows too high an infusion rate, resulting in accumulation; and curve C shows too low a rate, resulting in ineffective analgesia

Attempts have been made to calculate rates of infusion from individual drug pharmacokinetic data and using computer models, the idea being to produce satisfactory analgesia quickly and without risk of drug accumulation. Studies of the opioid drugs pethidine and alfentanil have produced guidelines for the infusion of these drugs. However, there remain several problems with these techniques.

- There is wide inter-individual variation in the plasma concentrations that produce effective analgesia. Calculations designed to produce a given plasma drug concentration will be ineffective in some patients whilst producing toxicity in others.

- Pharmacokinetically derived infusion rates will still produce widely different plasma drug concentrations in individual patients. In one study using pethidine it was found that the resulting plasma concentrations varied four-fold between patients.

- Increased vigilance is required when the rate of infusion is changed to avoid errors. When the rate requires adjustment several times over a short period there is an increased risk of incorrect rates being set.

Choices available for analgesic infusions

Route of drug administration

The standard approach uses the intravenous route. This provides direct access to the circulation and is not dependent upon any variability in drug absorption.

The subcutaneous route is an alternative in those patients requiring analgesia for whom maintenance of IV access is difficult. The technique involves the placement of fine gauge, short intravenous cannulae such as 23 G Y-Can (Wallace), which is made from Teflon, or a winged 23 G needle (Abbott) into the subcutaneous tissues (although the Teflon cannulae may kink they may be less likely to produce tissue inflammation). Positioning the cannula over the chest wall or abdomen can be particularly helpful since at these sites there will be minimal interference with the patient's activities. Appropriate infusion devices for this technique include the small, portable, battery-operated syringe drivers which encourage patient mobility.

When this route is used there may be considerable variability in the rate of drug absorption. Even after discontinuing the infusion there may be a depot of drug in the subcutaneous tissues to be absorbed. The rate of drug absorption is dependent upon the amount of fat present, which is poorly perfused with blood. Additionally, if the patient develops a low cardiac output the blood flow to the subcutaneous tissues will be further reduced. In such circumstances the analgesic drug will be poorly absorbed and pain will recur, resulting in peripheral vasoconstriction and a further decrease in drug absorption. During this time, drug continues to be deposited and when blood flow improves, toxic amounts of drug may be absorbed. Despite these difficulties this route has been used very successfully.

SETTING UP OPIOID INFUSIONS

Choice of drug

Several factors are important in making the decision about which drug should be used; they include the following:

Familiarity   Whenever opioid infusions are to be prescribed, the doctor and nursing staff who will be monitoring the patient should be familiar with the dosage, effects, and side-effects of the drug prescribed.

Availability   To be suitable for use by infusion the drug chosen should be available in an appropriate formulation. Subcutaneous infusions, for example, will require low-volume infusion rates. Diamorphine is particularly soluble in water and has high potency, therefore high concentrations can be given in a small volume, making it an appropriate choice for this route.

Pharmacological properties of the drug   Analgesics with a short duration of action are often recommended for use by infusion. With such drugs there will be a rapid reduction in effect once the infusion is reduced or discontinued. This would be particularly useful to provide rapid recovery from the adverse effects.

Lack of active metabolites   Some drugs have potentially toxic metabolites. For example the opioid drug pethidine is metabolized to norpethidine in the liver. This metabolite is a central nervous system stimulant and may accumulate when pethidine is given by continuous infusion, producing restlessness and irritability, particularly in patients with some degree of renal failure.

Adverse effects   Prolonged drug administration may be associated with an increased incidence of adverse effects. This may result from accumulation of the drug or of its metabolites. Analgesic agents with a low incidence of adverse effects would therefore be most appropriate for continuous infusion. All opioids will produce nausea and vomiting to some degree and when given by a continuous infusion, provision for the administration of antiemetic drugs regularly, or even added to the opioid infusion, must be made.

When to start an infusion

Patients in severe pain, those whose analgesic requirements are not met by the prescription of regular doses of opioid, and patients requiring intensive care who require frequent doses of analgesic agents may all benefit from a continuous infusion of an analgesic agent.

Suitable opioid drugs and infusion rates are shown in Table 9.1.

Table 9.1 Commonly used opioid infusion regimes

Drug	Infusion rates (adults)
Morphine	1-5 mg/h
Papaveretum	1-8 mg/h
Pethidine	10-50 mg/h
Fentanyl	50-150 μg/h

Requirements

IV access—preferably through an infusion line used solely for the analgesic drug. If other agents are being administered through the line check their compatibility.

Equipment—syringe pump and connecting tubing. If used with a Y-connector to an IV infusion this should ideally have a one-way valve.

Patient monitoring

A protocol should be developed with the nursing staff who will care for the patients. This should include the frequency and type of observations, details of drug prescribing, and safety instructions for all patients receiving opioid infusions. A separate chart should be available to facilitate regular recording of infusion rate, dose delivered, and patient observations, notably pulse, blood pressure, respiratory rate, and a simple assessment of the level of analgesia and sedation of the patient.

Guidelines should be agreed as to when to reduce or discontinue the infusion and also to adjustment of infusion rates if analgesia remains inadequate.

Details of the authors' hospital guidelines for the monitoring of patients with opioid infusions are shown in Fig. 9.2 and Table 9.2.

Difficulties with continuous infusions of opioids

- Drug accumulation may occur if the infusion is maintained at an unnecessarily high rate in the face of a changing clinical situation. This will be particularly evident if the patient's ability to eliminate the drug is changing. For example, the development of renal impairment in a patient receiving morphine may reduce the elimination of the active metabolites of morphine, resulting in toxicity.

- Infusion rates should be reduced in patients showing signs of impaired cardiovascular function or those who become hypovolaemic, perhaps as a consequence of continued postoperative bleeding. Liver blood flow in these patients may be reduced resulting in a consequent decrease in the rate of drug elimination.

- Mechanical failures or the incorrect setting of the equipment can lead to patients receiving too much or too little drug.

Disadvantages of continuous intravenous infusions

- Postoperative analgesic requirements vary widely between individuals and within individuals. For example, increased levels of pain will be experienced with movement, physiotherapy, and turning. A fixed-dose infusion may not be flexible enough to provide adequate analgesia in all these instances.

- The technique is more complex and there is greater scope for prescription and technical errors.

- The use of any infusion system requires careful clinical monitoring. The patients must be observed frequently so that the level of infusion can be adjusted to maintain good analgesia with minimum adverse effects.

- Nursing staff require additional training to ensure that they are familiar with the equipment and know how to check that it is functioning correctly.

Table 9.2 Monitoring patients receiving continuous opioid infusions

---

Postoperative analgesia—continuous-infusion pumps
The system must be initiated by the anaesthetist concerned.

Aim
To provide safe and reliable analgesia by means of a constant infusion using a syringe pump. Suitable infusions are:
Pethidine   600 mg in 60 ml (i.e. 10 mg/ml)
Omnopon   60 mg in 60 ml (i.e. 1 mg/ml)
Morphine   60 mg in 60 ml (i.e. 1 mg/ml).
Average dose required is 2-6 ml per hour.

Monitor and record
(1) pulse and blood pressure, as indicated surgically;
(2) pain score, 1 hourly;
(3) respiration rate, 1 hourly;
(4) pump setting (ml/h);
(5) amount of fluid remaining in syringe, hourly;
(6) nurse's initials.

Aim at
A pain score of 0-1, and a *responsive* patient at all times, i.e. a patient may be sleeping but should easily awake and respond to command.

Nursing actions
If patient is still in pain, increase rate by 1 ml/h.
If patient too sleepy, stop infusion for 1 h and then re-start at new rate 1 ml/h less than previous rate.
Call doctor if:
(1) patient is unrousable;
(2) if pain control is totally inadequate;
(3) if respiratory rate falls below 8 per min.

Medical actions
If patient unrousable, check airway and circulation. Stop infusion of analgesics until condition improves. Consider use of narcotic antagonist, e.g. naloxone 0.1 mg IV repeated as necessary.

If pain control is totally inadequate, give bolus of analgesic equal to current one-hour dose and review after 10 min. Consider further bolus injection if pain control still poor. When pain controlled, increase infusion rate by 1 ml/h above previous rate.

If respiratory rate is less than 8, stop infusion of narcotics and continue to review hourly until respiration rate is 8 or more. Then start infusion at half the previous rate.

CONTINUOUS ANALGESIA PUMP

Drug :– _____
For dilution details see prescription chart
[Add _____ mg to _____ ml of _____]

Dilution :– _____ mg/ml

Starting rate :– _____ ml/h

Range :– _____ to _____ ml/h

Name –

Hospital No. ....
Consultant ....

Pain Score (aim at 0 - 1)
  0 = none   1 = slight
  2 = significant   3 = severe

Call MO if:
  Pain not controlled
  Respiratory rate falls below 8
  Patient not easily rousable

Date –

Time	Pain Score	Respiration Rate	Pump Setting	Syringe Reading	Initials
1 am					
2					
3					
4					
5					
6 am					
7					
8					
9					
10					
11					
Noon					
1					
2					
3					
4					
5					
6 pm					
7					
8					
9					
10					
11					
MN					

Date –

Time	Pain Score	Respiration Rate	Pump Setting	Syringe Reading	Initials
1 am					
2					
3					
4					
5					
6 am					
7					
8					
9					
10					
11					
Noon					
1					
2					
3					
4					
5					
6 pm					
7					
8					
9					
10					
11					
MN					

Fig. 9.2 Hospital chart for monitoring patient with continuous analgesia pump

- Any equipment at the bedside which is capable of adjustment is open to abuse from the patients themselves or from relatives or visitors who may alter infusion rates. Ideally all infusion systems should have rate controls that are tamper-proof.

Alternative methods

Pharmaceutical companies have developed drug formulations to provide a slow, controlled release of drug from a depot given orally or applied topically. This endeavours to maintain a steady plasma concentration of drug similar to those seen with continuous intravenous infusions, throughout a prolonged period. Analgesic preparations that are available include both opioid drugs and some NSAIDs. Oral slow-release preparations include morphine, indomethacin, and diclofenac.

An experimental preparation of fentanyl available for controlled release following topical application is under investigation. It provides a given rate of drug delivery of 50–75 μg/h. There is a delay in onset of analgesic effects after application as drug is absorbed slowly from the depot through the skin. However, it appears to be useful in providing a background level of analgesia that may be increased by additional bolus doses of opioid.

Recent recommendations from the Committee of Safety of Medicine are that Papaveritum (Omnopon) should not be prescribed to women of childbearing potential.

10 Patient-controlled analgesia systems

The development and introduction of patient-controlled analgesia (PCA) systems into clinical practice has endeavoured to provide a method of analgesia which will bypass any difficulties relating to inappropriate dosing schedules, unpredictable drug absorption, or patient variability. It is a system that also avoids dependence upon the nurses or doctors to provide analgesic medication. These people may be unavailable at times or occupied with other tasks. Reliance upon them for analgesia may therefore be a factor in the failure of current regimes to provide satisfactory analgesia. With the PCA systems the patient is in control of his or her analgesia all the time. Not only does the PCA system provide improved analgesia; it also allows patients to have a positive behavioural control mechanism over their individual pain experiences.

This technique has been widely practised in midwifery for women in labour, initially with the use of nitrous oxide and air and currently with nitrous oxide in oxygen (Entonox). When this method is used for opioid administration, a reservoir of drug is maintained and a specifically designed infusion device allows a fixed quantity of drug to be administered in response to patient demand. These systems are most commonly used for the administration of opioid drugs by the intravenous route (which is discussed in this chapter) but they have also been used for epidural and subcutaneous routes of administration.

Safety features of the system include a lock-out interval setting (a time during which the system will remain unresponsive to additional patient demands). This can be adjusted to prevent the patient demanding an overdose of analgesic while still allowing the patient sufficient analgesic agent to control his or her pain. Should patients become sedated, their demands for analgesia will reduce, allowing recovery.

Since the early development of PCA systems, initially as a research tool and subsequently for clinical use, the equipment has been refined. The variants of the systems currently available are discussed below.

Bolus demand
This setting allows bolus doses of predetermined size to be delivered. The maximum amount of drug administered may be limited by the lock-out interval setting of the equipment or by further settings which limit the total dose of drug administered in a given time period.

Infusion demand
As an alternative to bolus demand the predetermined dose can be administered as a short infusion. This aims to reduce the incidence of side-effects which may be related to high plasma drug concentrations occurring after bolus doses.

Bolus demand and continuous infusion
A background infusion can be used to maintain analgesia with a facility for additional bolus doses available on demand. This may be a useful regimen for drugs with a short duration of action when plasma concentrations may decrease rapidly at times when the patient fails to make demands, for example while sleeping, and pain relief is inadequate on wakening. However, doubt remains as to its efficacy. Furthermore a background infusion may contribute to the development of acute drug tolerance without significantly improving analgesia. This method has sometimes been referred to as patient-augmented analgesia.

Bolus demand and variable infusion
This setting requires a more complicated, microprocessor-controlled infusion system which can alter the rate of background infusion depending upon the number of patient demands made for bolus doses. For example, a patient with inadequate analgesia will make frequent demands. The device will then set the background infusion at a higher rate. Similarly, it will reduce the rate of the background infusion when the patient is making infrequent demands.

The most commonly used systems in clinical practice are the *bolus* demand systems with or without the facility for a constant background infusion. Two commonly used PCA systems in the

UK are the *Graseby PCAS* and the *Abbott Lifecare PCAS*. Both systems allow for bolus demands with or without a background infusion and have variable rates allowing the boluses to be administered as infusions.

Pattern of patient demands

The typical pattern of bolus demands made by patients using a PCA system shows a high rate initially—providing a loading dose—followed by a more stable period of maintenance demands. However, there may be periods of less frequent demands such as during sleep, which may be followed by periods of catching up with increased demands. Periods of increased demand for improved analgesia may be associated with physiotherapy, mobilization, and other nursing procedures.

Setting up a PCA system

Prescription variables:

1. Choice of drug   Experimental studies have shown that PCA systems have been successful with a number of different opioids for relieving acute pain. The most commonly used drug is morphine. Other useful opioids are pethidine and papaveretum.

The ideal analgesic drug for use in PCA systems would have a rapid onset of action with an intermediate duration of action to enhance the control of analgesia. A low incidence of side-effects and a lack of drug interactions would be advantageous. The most widely used opioids in PCA systems are morphine and pethidine. The duration of action of buprenorphine and methadone may be too long for them to gain widespread favour whilst fentanyl and its analogues may be too short acting. These latter drugs may benefit from combined low-dose background infusions with additional bolus-demand facilities. Recent studies have used oxymorphone and hydromorphone after Caesarian section and have shown that these drugs are useful alternatives for use in PCA systems.

Agonist–antagonist opioid drugs exhibit a ceiling effect to their analgesia and respiratory-depressant effects. These drugs may therefore be useful alternatives for use in PCA systems with a reduced risk of respiratory depression.

2. Size of dose The choice of bolus dose size should be that drug dose which will produce analgesia with low incidence of side-effects. In adults, a bolus dose of 1 mg of morphine is an effective bolus dose. A lower dose produces inadequate analgesia whilst doses of 2 mg are associated, in some patients, with a higher incidence of respiratory depression. Studies of PCA systems in children have used bolus doses calculated on an individual basis from body weight.

3. Dose rate Most PCA systems will allow for a choice in the rate of administration of the bolus dose of the drug.

4. Lock-out interval The lock-out time interval needs to be short enough to allow the patient to administer the drug at high initial rates soon after starting the system, but not so short as to allow overdosage later. The time interval should also take into account the time taken for each bolus dose to prove effective. With too short a time interval, demands may be made before doses previously given have been effective, leading to overdosage. The most commonly used time intervals are of the range 5–10 min.

5. Background infusion rate The concept of the use of a background infusion appears theoretically sound. However, it has been suggested that there appears to be little benefit in analgesia over a simple bolus system alone. The use of an infusion merely increases the quantities of analgesic agent given without improving analgesia.

6. Maximum dose rate Some devices available for self administration of opioids have a facility for setting a maximum dose rate. This may be as a maximum amount of drug per hour or each four-hour period. This will provide a further safety feature and should allow the use of shorter lock-out periods since this feature would allow only a fixed maximum amount of drug per given time.

Table 10.1 lists some opioid drugs and doses which have been used in PCA systems to provide analgesia for acute pain.

Table 10.1   Guidelines for bolus doses and lock-out intervals
using opioids in PCA systems

Opioid	Bolus dose (mg)	Lock-out time interval (mg)
Morphine	0.5–3	5–20
Pethidine	5–30	5–15
Fentanyl	0.02–0.1	3–10
Methadone	0.5–3	10–20
Nalbuphine	1–5	5–15
Buprenorphine	0.03–0.2	10–20
Hydromorphone	0.1–0.6	5–15
Oxymorphone	0.1–0.6	5–15

Patient monitoring

Table 10.2 gives details of the schedule in use in the authors
hospital for monitoring patients receiving intravenous opioids
from PCA systems. Figure 10.1 shows the chart used to record
the results of patient monitoring.

With all patients in pain the monitoring must include an assessment of the patient's pain. Methods and rating scales have been
discussed in Chapter 2. Simple methods are useful for continuous
assessment and problem patients should be easily identified.

Procedures to be followed in patients with inadequate pain
control or those with unwanted or dangerous drug effects must be
detailed.

In addition, schedules should record the prescribed settings for
the PCA system and checks on drug administration to ensure that
the equipment is functioning correctly.

Hazards associated with PCA systems

Although the use of the patient as his or her own control to
regulate the administration of drug is a safety feature of the PCA
system, there remain hazards through their incorrect use. These
may occur from a number of errors.

Prescription errors

- Inappropriate demand dose.
- Incorrect lock-out interval.
- High background infusion.

Provision errors

- Incorrect drug concentration prepared.
- Accidental drug administration—this can occur when new syringes are connected, or when partially empty syringes are removed. At such times the infusion line should be disconnected or cross clamped prior to these manoeuvres.

Absent or incorrectly placed one-way valves in the infusion system may affect the amount of drug administered, with the analgesic being diverted into reservoir bags of intravenous fluids or other drugs administered through the same intravenous line.

Syringes which are not correctly placed within the infusion system can administer excessive drug doses due to siphoning of the drug from the syringe. The Abbott system manufacturers have developed purpose designed tubing for connecting to their PCA system which includes an anti-siphon device to prevent this occurring. (Fig. 10.2)

Patient factors

Failure to understand the PCA system should not occur because patients should be assessed for their suitability and the system should be properly explained, preoperatively. With most patients, such a problem can be overcome by careful instruction and discussion of the benefits of the system, although there may remain patients who cannot be sufficiently well motivated to use the system.

Intentional abuse may occur in patients who are generally susceptible to the mood elevating effects of the opioid analgesics. It does appear to be a very rare hazard.

Initiation of demands by people other than the patient has been reported to have occurred when nurses gave additional boluses for

PATIENT-CONTROLLED ANALGESIA PUMP

Drug :- _____

For dilution details see prescription chart

[Add _____ mg to _____ ml of _____]

Pump setting

Loading dose _____

Bolus _____

Dose duration _____

Lockout _____

Concentration _____

Background _____

Initial any changes

Name –

Hospital No. ....

Consultant ....

Pain Score (aim at 0 - 1)

0 = none   1 = slight

2 = significant   3 = severe

Call MO if:

Pain not controlled

Respiratory rate falls below 8

Patient not easily rousable

Date –

Time	Pain Score	Respiration Rate	Pump Setting	Syringe Reading	Initials
1 am					
2					
3					
4					
5					
6 am					
7					
8					
9					
10					
11					
Noon					
1					
2					
3					
4					
5					
6 pm					
7					
8					
9					
10					
11					
MN					

Date –

Time	Pain Score	Respiration Rate	Pump Setting	Syringe Reading	Initials
1 am					
2					
3					
4					
5					
6 am					
7					
8					
9					
10					
11					
Noon					
1					
2					
3					
4					
5					
6 pm					
7					
8					
9					
10					
11					
MN					

Fig. 10.1 Hospital chart for monitoring patient using patient-controlled analgesia pump

Table 10.2   Monitoring patients using PCA systems

Postoperative analgesia. Patient-controlled analgesia pumps

The system must be initiated by the anaesthetist concerned.

Suitable infusions are:
Pethidine   600 mg in 60 ml i.e. 10 mg/ml
Omnopon   60 mg in 60 ml i.e. 1 mg/ml
Morphine   60 mg in 60 ml i.e. 1 mg/ml.
Average dose required is 2-6 ml per hour.

Monitor and record
(1) pulse and blood pressure, as indicated surgically;
(2) pain score, 1 hourly;
(3) respiration rate, 1 hourly;
(4) total mg infused;
(5) amount of fluid remaining in syringe, hourly;
(6) nurse's initials.

Aim at
A pain score of 0-1, and a *responsive* patient at all times, i.e. a patient may be sleeping but should easily awake and respond to command.

Nursing actions
If patient is still in pain, is he using the demand button properly? Give instructions.
Call doctor if:
(1) patient is too sleepy;
(2) pain control is totally inadequate;
(3) respiratory rate falls below 8 per min.

Medical actions
If patient is too sleepy, turn off any background infusion.
    If patient unrousable, check airway and circulation. Stop infusion of analgesics until condition improves. Consider use of narcotic antagonist, e.g. naloxone, 0.1 mg IV repeated as necessary.
    If pain control is totally inadequate, check that the patient is receiving boluses when the button is pressed. Check that the lock-out time is reasonable (10-20 min). Consider increasing the size of the bolus dose.
    If respiratory rate is less than 8, remove demand button from patient and stop any background infusion. Continue to review hourly until respiration rate is 8 or more. Then return button to patient.
    If there are continuing problems, contact the duty anaesthetist for advice.

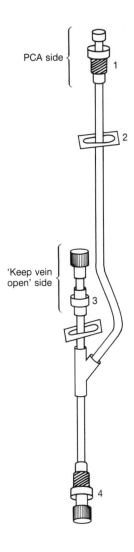

Fig. 10.2 Abbott PCA infusion set (No 3559). 1, anti-siphon valve; 2, slide clamp; 3, back-check valve; 4, secure lock and male adaptor

patients. We have known additional boluses to be administered by a relative, resulting in excessive sedation.

Equipment malfunction

Excess or inadequate drug administration may occur with equipment failure.

Syringes may empty at faster or slower rates than programmed if incorrect sizes or specifications of syringes are used in individual PCA systems.

Inadequate analgesia with PCA systems

When the degree of pain relief patients obtain using PCA systems is assessed, it is noteworthy that often patients do not administer sufficient analgesia to completely abolish their pain despite the ability to do so. The reasons for this are complex. Patients may not envisage complete analgesia as being possible, or there may be failure to understand the system or fear of the adverse effects of the drugs administered. In addition, staff may encourage caution, discouraging patients from making demands unless really necessary or to 'be careful not to use too much'. Even when all of these difficulties have been excluded patients still do not relieve their pain completely. It may be that a small amount of pain, sufficient to cause discomfort but not distress, is necessary to protect the patient from harm. Alternatively a minor degree of discomfort may be preferable to the unwanted effects of the drug.

Psychological factors

The degree of pain tolerated by patients will vary enormously. It will depend upon various psychological and social factors. In addition, the patient's personality and other psychological factors may be a reason for the patient aiming at a tolerable level of pain rather than complete analgesia. This may include the general feeling that a *need to suffer* is part of the healing process.

Inadequate analgesia may also result from practical errors in the use of the PCA system, including the following.

Incorrect prescriptions

A prescription for too small or infrequent doses of the analgesic drug being used is an obvious cause of failure. In addition, unnecessarily large doses may be prescribed, leading to unpleasant side-effects. As a consequence the patient may prefer to suffer the pain rather than the adverse effects of the drug.

Equipment failure

Problems with the pump or its connections can result in excessive or reduced drug administration. Connections of the equipment should be routinely checked and the levels of drug remaining in the reservoir or syringe recorded, allowing a further check on the amount of drug that the machine has delivered.

Shared intravenous access

PCA systems should not share intravenous access sites with other infusion lines without a one-way valve being incorporated into each solution-delivery set. If the PCA system is connected to an intravenous access site without a one-way valve it is possible for the pump to direct the analgesic agent into the tubing and reservoir of the IV bag. This will result in inadequate analgesia with an additional risk of the drug being administered in a large bolus from the other IV infusion if this is then given quickly.

Uses of PCA systems

Clinical

Postoperative pain   PCA systems are being increasingly used in hospitals for the management of postoperative pain. They are principally used for patients undergoing major surgery although increased availability of the equipment may allow their wider use.

Obstetrics   The technique was first used to provide analgesia for women in labour using nitrous oxide, originally in air and now in oxygen. Intravenous opioids are now used both in labour and to provide postoperative analgesia following Caesarian section deliveries.

Trauma   The PCA system offers the advantage of good pain control with avoidance of excessive sedation.

Burns   Patients require analgesia not only for their thermal injury but will also experience increased requirements for pain control during procedures such as wound cleaning and changes of dressing. Using standard methods of analgesic administration this could be covered if additional bolus doses were administered prior to these procedures. However, patients will vary in the amount of drug required, not only between individuals, but also in the same patient at different times during recovery. Even using this regime patients will still not receive sufficient analgesia for these procedures. Therefore allowing patients access to a PCA system will enable self-administration of analgesia to appropriate levels which allow them comfort during the procedures.

Paediatrics The youngest reported patient in whom this system has been used successfully was six years old. In that study the system used a background infusion rate and bolus doses. The doses were calculated on an individual basis for both the infusion rate and for the bolus administration. However, problems were seen in one child when the nursing staff administered additional boluses of analgesic to a child who seemed to be in pain. This resulted in excessive sedation, fortunately with no serious sequelae.

Terminal care PCA systems can be used in hospital for the management of acute exacerbations of the patient's pain or worsening of the clinical condition. They are also finding use in ambulatory patients—a particular benefit being the ability to administer epidural opioids by the PCA apparatus, for longer-term pain control.

Research

PCA systems are widely used in the assessment of new analgesic agents. In the management of acute pain, patients can be given the new analgesic drug or a placebo while also allowing them access to a PCA system with a conventional opioid such as morphine, to provide analgesia on demand. The efficacy of the new agent can then be compared with the placebo effect by looking at the reductions in the amount of morphine required to provide analgesia in the two groups—the so-called 'morphine sparing' effect.

Similarly it can be used to compare the efficacy of preoperative psychological preparation in improving postoperative analgesia by comparing morphine requirements in the different groups.

DISADVANTAGES OF THE PCA SYSTEMS

Cost

The initial cost of equipment for this technique is high. At present, PCA systems cost in the region of £2000 ($3500). To provide these systems for every patient in acute pain who may benefit would require a large capital outlay. Evidence of cost saving as a result of using PCA systems can only be envisaged in terms of a reduction in nursing time spent in duties relating to the provision of analgesia for the patients, allowing more time for other patient needs. Improvement in analgesia may also benefit by reducing morbidity and length of hospital stay and thereby providing cost savings.

Monitoring

Although these systems have an inherent safety feature in that the patients themselves make the demands it is easy to over-estimate the safety and become complacent. The use of these techniques does not obviate the need for close monitoring of the patients or vigilance in observing side-effects of the drugs used. Reports of both nursing staff and relatives administering unnecessary analgesic drug boluses for patients may be few, but they indicate that the present systems must be monitored.

11 Epidural and intrathecal opioids

Experiments in animals have demonstrated the effect of small doses of opioid drugs on nociceptive transmission at the spinal cord level. Transmission of impulses from noxious stimuli upwards to the brain was inhibited. When chronic spinal catheterization was performed in animals it was shown that intrathecal administration of opioids could produce significant and long-lasting increases in nociceptive thresholds using thermal, electrical, and mechanical pain stimuli.

Spinal effects of opioid drugs result from alterations in pain transmission at the level of the first- and second-order neurons in the dorsal grey matter. Receptors for the opioid drugs are located in the substantia gelatinosa in the vicinity of the primary afferent terminals. The specific binding sites are believed to be pre-synaptic, with the actions resulting from inhibition of transmitter release specific to nociceptive transmission.

When used in humans, the benefits of epidural or intrathecal opioid analgesia compared with that produced by local anaesthetic agents administered by the same routes include the achievement of analgesia without sensory or motor deficit and, as a result of the lack of autonomic blockade, analgesia without the risks of hypotension. In addition, lower doses of opioid drugs are used when these routes are employed and as a result, there is a low incidence of respiratory depression.

Factors influencing the action of intrathecal and epidural opioids

Lipid solubility The degree of lipid solubility of the agent determines the rate of penetration through lipid membranes and this will influence the onset of analgesia. The most lipid-soluble drugs (for example fentanyl) will have a quicker onset of analgesia as a result of more rapid penetration into the neural tissue and their sites of action. However, the duration of action will be reduced as these drugs will be most rapidly cleared after absorption into the blood vessels. The slow onset of analgesia with a less lipid-soluble drug such as morphine is thought to be related to slow penetration into the spinal cord and sequestration of drug in the cerebro-spinal fluid (CSF).

Elimination   The duration of effects of the drugs will be influenced by the rate at which they are cleared from their sites of action. The endogenous opioid peptides are rapidly metabolized by peptidase enzymes in the CSF; exogenous opioid drugs are normally eliminated after absorption into the blood.

Route of administration

Drugs administered by the epidural route must penetrate the dura in addition to passing through the neural tissue, resulting in a delayed onset of action. Drugs may be absorbed from the epidural site into the fat normally present in this region and from there eliminated via the epidural venous plexus. Higher plasma concentrations are achieved after epidural administration compared to the intrathecal route.

Unwanted effects

Central nervous sytem effects   The typical central nervous system effects of opioids—euphoria, sedation, and respiratory depression—still occur when these routes are used. This has been taken as evidence that opioids, when administered intrathecally or epidurally, reach higher centres. This may be the result of drug redistribution by the blood following absorption from the CSF or as a result of bulk flow within the CSF.

Early central nervous system effects are thought to result from drug distribution after vascular uptake, whereas the late effects may result from CSF transfer. Late effects are most commonly seen with morphine which, because of its low lipid solubility, persists in the CSF in appreciable quantity.

Peripheral effects   Pruritis occurs after both epidural and intrathecal administration, although widely differing rates have been reported. Some studies have reported this complication occurring in up to two thirds of the patients who have received morphine. Itching is also associated with fentanyl, diamorphine, and pethidine administration, although the incidence is lower than with morphine. Itching is unrelated to histamine release or to the dose of drug used. It is usually unrelated to the segmental area of action of the opioid drug and occurs frequently around the head and neck. It may be severe and prolonged and may last up to 30 h after morphine administration. Pruritis may be relieved by the systemic administration of small doses of naloxone (0.1 mg) without adversely affecting analgesia.

Nausea and vomiting are associated with the use of opioids whatever route is employed. The incidence after epidural and intrathecal administration is between 30 and 50 per cent.

Urinary retention is variable with an incidence of 30–40 per cent. It occurs more commonly in males and is increased after intrathecal compared with epidural administration. The mechanism by which this occurs is unclear. Since minimal effects on bladder function are seen after systemic opioid use, this adverse effect must be due to the high concentrations produced around the spinal cord, affecting bladder-control mechanisms. The effects may be prolonged, up to 14–16 h, although they may be relieved by systemic administration of naloxone.

Respiratory depression after epidural and intrathecal opioids

Respiratory depression is a major concern when intrathecal and epidural opioids are used. It is of particular concern since it may occur some time (up to 24 h) after the drug has been given (see Table 11.1). There appear to be several groups of patients who are at increased risk—elderly patients and patients who have received systemic opioids or other central nervous system depressant drugs (such as benzodiazepines). The less lipid-soluble opioids are most prone to this complication since a large reservoir of drug remains in the CSF and may be distributed to higher centres. Administration of opioid into the epidural space in the thoracic region or intrathecal administration also appears to increase the risk. Large doses by either route will further increase the risks of this complication.

Naloxone will reverse the respiratory depression but repeated doses or infusions may be required for the prolonged period during which the patient remains at risk following intrathecal and epidural administration.

Table 11.1 Incidence of respiratory depression after epidural opioids

Drug	Dose (mg)	Time occurring
Morphine	2–10	4–22 h
Diamorphine	2–10	20 min–4.5 h
Pethidine	50–100	5–30 min
Methadone	4–6	20 min–4 h
Fentanyl	0.1 μg	30 min–4 h

Adapted from Morgan 1989.

Disadvantages

The nature and incidence of unwanted effects after epidural and intrathecal administration of opioids remain the major factors limiting the use of these techniques. The most serious complication is respiratory depression, although the minor sequelae of pruritus, nausea and vomiting, and urinary retention are common and distressing.

Indications and uses of epidural opioids

- Postoperative pain—used to provide analgesia after thoracic, upper, and lower abdominal surgery and also after orthopaedic procedures on the lower limbs.
- Obstetrics—epidural opioids have been used to provide analgesia after Caesarian section operations and also to provide analgesia in labour. Small doses of fentanyl will reduce the requirements for epidural local analgesic agents during the first stage of labour.
- Trauma—analgesia for rib fractures and limb injuries can be provided very successfully using epidural opioids.

Drugs and administration

The ideal agent for spinal use should have

- high lipid solubility, which will produce rapid passage of the drug through the dura, permitting epidural use. High lipid solubility will enable rapid absorption of the drug from the spinal depot and reduce the risks of delayed respiratory depression;

- high affinity for the μ receptor;
- high efficacy;
- rapid metabolism—to minimize systemic accumulation and reduce the risk of systemic side-effects.

Epidural opioid infusions

Continuous infusions may be used to provide prolonged analgesia with the use of shorter-acting opioids such as fentanyl and alfentanil. Morphine has also been used in infusions for post-operative pain and the use of patient-controlled analgesia systems have also been reported with epidural opioids.

Currently used drugs

The dose range of drugs administered by this route is shown in Table 11.2.

Table 11.2 Commonly used opioids for epidural administration

Drug	Dose range (mg)
Pethidine	25–100
Morphine	0.1–10
Diamorphine	0.5–10
Fentanyl	0.1–0.2
Methadone	4–6
Buprenorphine	0.06–0.3
Phenoperidine	2
Meptazinol	30–90

Adapted from Morgan 1989.

Morphine
Intrathecal administration of morphine is associated with a more rapid onset of action than after epidural use. The duration of

action after intrathecal administration is also longer than after epidural administration with analgesia lasting for up to 24 h. After epidural administration the analgesia produced by morphine lasts for 8–12 h. Morphine preparations for epidural and spinal use should be preservative free. The usual preparations of morphine found on the ward contain a preservative, sodium metabisulphite, which may be neurotoxic.

Doses: Intrathecal 0.5–1 mg
           Epidural   2–5 mg.

Diamorphine

This drug has a more rapid onset of analgesia when administered epidurally in comparison with morphine. It has also been used intrathecally to provide prolonged analgesia. In addition it is available as a freeze-dried preparation and therefore contains no preservative.

Doses: Intrathecal 0.5–1 mg
           Epidural   1–5 mg.

Fentanyl

This is the safest and most reliable agent currently used but analgesia is of relatively short duration—approximately 2–3 h. To counter this short duration of action it has been given by continuous infusion into epidural catheters.

Doses: Epidural—bolus 80–100 μg
           —continuous infusion up to 75 μg/h.

Novel spinal analgesic agents

Clonidine

This is an α_2-adrenergic receptor agonist drug which is primarily used in the treatment of hypertension. However, when applied epidurally or spinally in experimental animals, this drug also produces analgesia.

The analgesic effects are believed to result from pre- and post-synaptic α_2-receptor activation in the spinal cord which may block pain transmission by inhibiting the release of the transmitter substance P and by reducing the activity of dorsal horn neurons.

Midazolam

Midazolam is a water-soluble benzodiazepine drug generally used for sedation and anaesthesia. In experimental animals it has also been shown to produce spinally mediated analgesic effects.

The role of intrathecal opioids

The risk of respiratory depression and the incidence of complications are higher after intrathecal opioid administration. It is likely that at present this route will be little used for patients other than those who are in a high dependency or intensive care area.

Currently, epidural morphine and fentanyl are the most commonly used agents. Several workers have addressed the safety aspects of the use of these agents by this route and guidelines are reported below.

Guidelines for the safe use of intrathecal and epidural opioids in acute pain

Recent guidelines suggested from an acute pain service in the USA are listed below (Ready, L.B. and Edwards, W.T. (1990). *Anesthesiology*, 72, 213). (Reproduced with permission of the Editor and Publishers.)

1. Careful patient selection with modification of opioid doses for patient age and physical status.
2. Regular follow up by skilled and knowledgeable physicians.
3. Sound education of all nursing personnel regarding the use and risks of intraspinal opioids including instruction in bedside monitoring techniques which ensure early detection of respiratory depression.
4. Provision for periodic nursing updates.
5. The use of printed protocols and standard orders developed jointly by physicians and nurses to govern the use of intraspinal narcotics including those permitting immediate intervention by nurses, if necessary.

6. Provision of a support system within the hospital which is capable of providing immediate airway management and ventilatory support at all times.

7. Continuing quality assurance review of all problems.

These authors believe, with adherence to these principles for safe administration, that intraspinal opioids may be as safe as intramuscular injections on hospital wards.

12 Inflammation and non-steroidal anti-inflammatory drugs

Peripheral mechanisms of inflammatory pain revolve around the sensitization of nociceptors by prostaglandins, particularly prostaglandin E2 (PGE2) and prostacyclin. These increase the pain response to other chemical mediators such as histamine and bradykinin, which are released in response to cell damage from trauma. The characteristic signs of inflammation are described as 'rubor, dolor, and tumor'—erythema, pain, and swelling—and result from the effects of these mediators on peripheral vessels. These substances produce vasodilatation (rubor), nociception (resulting in pain), and increased capillary permeability (resulting in swelling).

The analgesic and anti-inflammatory properties of some plant extracts (now recognized as containing salicylates) have been known from earliest times. Records of their uses have been found in Egyptian papyri and they were widely used in early Roman and Greek medicine.

The nineteenth century saw the preparation of salicylic acid, initially from natural sources and later from chemical synthesis. The preparation of aspirin (acetyl salicylic acid) was documented in 1853 by Charles Gerhardt, Professor of Chemistry in Strasbourg, but its full commercial exploitation did not occur for some 40 years. Early investigators using salicylates recognized the gastric irritant effects and also that this could be relieved by the administration of sodium bicarbonate. High doses of salicylates were employed therapeutically in the management of acute rheumatic illnesses and nausea, vomiting, and tinnitus, due to toxicity, were common side-effects. The early physician's therapeutic indications for these agents recognized their analgesic, antipyretic, and anti-inflammatory effects.

Salicylates are probably the most well recognized of drugs that now fall into the category of mild analgesics with anti-inflammatory activity classed as non-steroidal anti-inflammatory agents

(NSAIDs). The chemical classes of drugs in this group are widely different; however, their actions can be grouped overall as

- analgesia;
- antipyretic;
- anti-inflammatory.

Generally all agents will have analgesic effects but there may be considerable variations in their anti-inflammatory activity.

These agents predominantly act peripherally at the site of injury rather than in the central nervous system where opioid drugs principally act. They inhibit cyclo-oxygenase dependent prostaglandin synthesis. Some actions of NSAIDs may result from prostaglandin inhibition within the central nervous system. Prostaglandins are released in almost all forms of tissue damage and are thought to sensitize the pain receptors to different stimuli such as chemical mediators, heat and mechanical stimuli. Chemical mediators released during the inflammatory process will interact and produce pain at lower concentrations as a result of this prior sensitization (see Fig. 12.1).

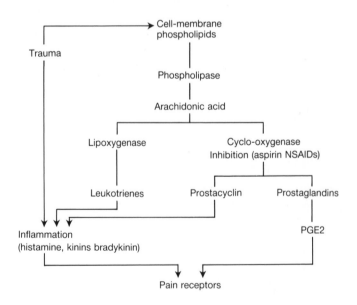

Fig. 12.1 Mechanism of prostaglandin inhibition by NSAIDs

When used as analgesics these agents all exhibit a ceiling effect—a dose beyond which further improvements in analgesia will not occur. They are also less likely to produce sedation, respiratory depression, or mood changes.

They are widely used in the control of minor or moderate pain, headache, toothache, and low back pain for example. When used for musculoskeletal disorders both their analgesic and anti-inflammatory actions are useful. For postoperative pain they have been found to be particularly useful after dental surgery, for example after extraction of wisdom teeth, and parenteral preparations have also been used to provide analgesia after some orthopaedic operations such as hip replacement. It is thought that their administration preoperatively would inhibit prostaglandin synthesis prior to the tissue disruption of surgery and thereby reduce the requirement for postoperative analgesia, but this remains speculative.

Adverse effects

The adverse effects of these agents include the following.

Gastrointestinal effects

These are the most frequently reported side effects of non steroidal anti-inflammatory drugs. Gastric irritation, dyspepsia, and ulceration, often leading to upper-gastrointestinal haemorrhage, have occurred. To reduce the incidence of these problems they can be prescribed in combination with H_2-receptor blocking drugs (cimetidine). Diarrhoea and constipation have also been reported.

Fluid balance

These agents produce sodium and water retention, which may lead to cardiac failure in patients with poor myocardial function. They reduce renal blood flow and lead to a reduction in urine production.

Renal tract

Combinations of aspirin and phenacetin were well recognized causes of renal failure—the so-called 'analgesic nephropathy'. Interstitial nephritis as a cause of impaired renal function has also been associated with modern NSAID therapy. Patients at particular risk of renal damage are those who may have impaired renal function or reduced renal perfusion, such as patients with cardiac failure, shock, or patients requiring intensive care.

Hypersensitivity

Acute bronchospasm, urticaria, and oedema can occur following ingestion of NSAIDs in sensitive patients. This was first recognized with aspirin. These patients generally have a history of asthma and frequently have nasal polyps.

Haematological effects

These agents reduce platelet aggregation. This reduction in platelet 'stickiness' has been used therapeutically in the prevention of cerebrovascular accidents and myocardial infarction using low-dose aspirin. Bone marrow suppression, with agranulocytosis, pancytopaenia, and aplastic anaemia have occurred with several different agents.

Idiosyncratic reactions

Other more unusual reactions to these agents can occur, including rashes and photosensitivity.

Classes of NSAIDs

There are numerous NSAIDs available. Examples of agents from differing chemical classes are described. For individual drug dosages see Table 12.1.

Salicylates—aspirin

Originally the drug of first choice for mild pain, headache, musculoskeletal, or arthritic pain. More modern NSAIDs may now be used for some indications as they may be better tolerated. Aspirin is contra-indicated in children under 12 years because of its links with Reyes syndrome (a severe illness with high mortality from coma and hepatic failure) except for specific clinical condi-

Table 12.1 Doses of commonly used non-steroidal anti-inflammatory drugs

Drug	Usual total daily dose (mg)	Usual single dose (mg)	Usual dose interval (h)	Time to peak effect (h)
Aspirin	1800-3600	300-600	4	0.25
Diclofenac	75-150	75	8	1-3
Fenoprofen	1800-2400	600	6-8	1-2
Ibuprofen	1200-2400	300-600	6-8	0.5-1.5
Indomethacin	75-150	25-50	6-12	1-2
Ketoprofen	100-200	25-50	6-8	0.5-2
Naproxen	500-750	250	12	1-2
Paracetamol	2000-4000	500-1000	4	1
Phenylbutazone	300-400	100	6-8	2
Piroxicam	20-30	10-20	12-24	2

tions such as juvenile arthritis. There is little anti-inflammatory activity, in adults, with doses less than 3 g daily.

Aspirin has been marketed in numerous formulations in attempts to reduce the gastrointestinal side-effect, which remains the most common reason for discontinuing treatment.

Cyclic acetic acid—indomethacin
This drug may be used for pain and moderate to severe inflammation in acute musculoskeletal disorders, and is particularly useful in acute gout. However, its use is associated with a high incidence of adverse effects, notably dizziness, headaches, and gastrointestinal disturbances. Slow-release formulations and suppositories are available and oral doses should be taken with food.

Aryl acetic acids—diclofenac
This drug is available as an oral sustained-release preparation, as suppository, and also as a parenteral preparation for intramuscular administration. In its parenteral form it has been advocated as suitable for the relief of pain from renal colic or for postoperative pain on its own or in addition to opioids.

Proprionic acid derivatives—ibuprofen

This is the most widely used agent of this group. As an oral preparation, it is used in mild pain of musculoskeletal type. It has a lower incidence of side-effects compared with other NSAIDs but it has only weak anti-inflammatory action. Other agents in this group include **naproxen**, **fenoprofen**, and **ketoprofen**.

Fenamates—mefenamic acid

This drug is related to indomethacin and is useful in mild to moderate pain. It has little anti-inflammatory effect and should be administered after food.

Oxicams—piroxicam

This drug has the benefit of good efficacy with a prolonged duration of action allowing a once-daily dosage schedule. It has a greater incidence of adverse effects than ibuprofen, particularly in the elderly.

p-Amino phenols—paracetamol

This drug is unusual among the NSAIDs as its action is generally believed to result from the inhibition of prostaglandin production within the central nervous system. It is the most commonly used analgesic agent and is first-line agent for the management of mild and moderate pain. It has replaced aspirin as the analgesic and antipyretic agent of choice in children. It is usually administered orally although suppository preparations are available. Gastro-intestinal side effects are minimal and the risks of renal and hepatic damage are limited to overdose.

Doses:

Adults	0.5–1 g orally, 4–6 hourly
	0.5–1 g suppository, 4–6 hourly.
Children	10–15 mg/kg orally, 4–6 hourly
	15–20 mg/kg suppository, 4–6 hourly.

13 Pharmacology of local anaesthetic agents

Local anaesthetic agents produce a transient inhibition of nerve impulse conduction. Normally when a nerve transmits an impulse its permeability to sodium is increased, resulting in a change in the electrical state of the cell (depolarization). When local anaesthetics are used the permeability of the cell membrane to sodium is reduced. This results in a slow rate of rise of the depolarization potential and failure to achieve the critical threshold for the propagation of the electrical change (action potential). Local anaesthetics can be used to block the transmission of painful stimuli at any point from the peripheral nerve to the spinal cord.

The basic chemical structures of the local anaesthetic agents in current use are shown in Fig. 13.1.

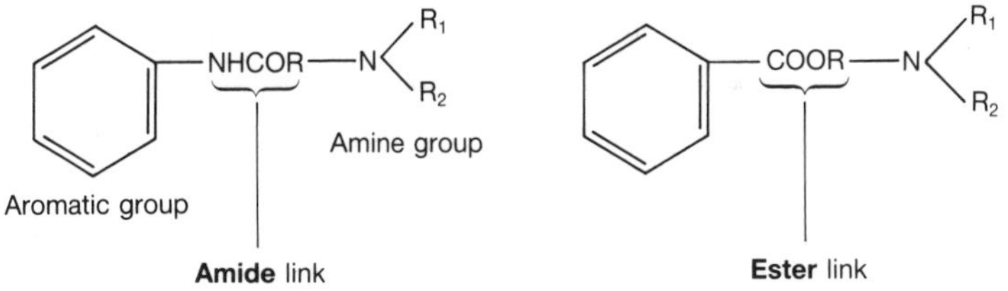

Fig. 13.1 Chemical structure of local anaesthetic agents

The local-anaesthetic module includes an aromatic and an amine terminal with intermediate chain. They are generally classified according to the chemical nature of the linkage group between the aromatic portion and the intermediate chain structure of the molecule. This group may be an amide or an ester. Amide-linked anaesthetics are generally more stable and are metabolized in the liver. Ester-linked agents are hydrolysed in the plasma.

Changes in the chemical structure of the molecules alter the physicochemical properties of the local anaesthetic agent and change the profile of the local anaesthetic activity.

Local anaesthetic agents are weak bases. At the pH of tissues the agents exist in both unionized and ionized forms. Only the unionized form which is lipid soluble will be able to penetrate the cell membranes. The degree of lipid solubility of the agent is therefore important in determining drug potency. The local anaesthetic base is relatively insoluble in water and so is generally prepared as the hydrochloride salt or as the carbonate form, the latter having a more rapid onset. Examples of commonly used local anaesthetic agents are listed in Table 13.1.

Table 13.1   Commonly used local
anaesthetic agents

Local anaesthetic	Chemical structure
Lignocaine	Amide
Bupivacaine	Amide
Prilocaine	Amide
Procaine	Ester
Amethocaine	Ester

Local anaesthetic agents

Lignocaine

Lignocaine has become the most widely used local anaesthetic agent. It has good powers of penetration and can be used topically, for infiltration as well as for regional blocks in appropriate concentrations. In addition, by virtue of its membrane-stabilizing effects, it has proved successful in the treatment of ventricular dysrhythmias.

Prilocaine

Prilocaine is more slowly absorbed than lignocaine and so is less dependent upon the addition of vasoconstrictor agents. It has a lower acute toxicity on the central nervous system and is rapidly metabolized in the liver. Side-effects include the development of methaemoglobinaemia after high doses of the drug, which should be treated with intravenous injection of methylene blue (2 mg/kg).

Bupivacaine

Bupivacaine is a more potent local anaesthetic drug and has similarly increased toxicity. It has a prolonged duration of local anaesthetic action. The addition of adrenalin as a vasoconstrictor has minimal effects on the duration of action or toxicity.

Cocaine

This was one of the earliest local anaesthetic agents but is now rarely used therapeutically. It is an effective surface local anaesthetic with marked vasoconstrictor properties, but has now been superseded by less toxic drugs. It is still used in otolaryngology (ENT surgery) to produce topical local anaesthesia in the nasal airways where its vasoconstrictor effects will reduce bleeding at operation. For topical analgesia in other areas, toxic effects including central nervous system stimulation with excitation, tachycardia, and hypertension preclude its use.

Ropivacaine

This agent is a newly developed amide local anaesthetic which is a congener of mepivacaine and bupivacaine. In clinical studies it appears to have sensory and motor effects that are similar in duration to bupivacaine, and similar potency. However, in human studies, its clearance after intravenous administration is more rapid than that of bupivacaine, and it is also less cardiotoxic, making it a safer agent.

EMLA cream

This preparation—a 'eutectic mixture of local anaesthetic'— includes prilocaine and lignocaine and has been developed as a local anaesthetic for intact skin. It is applied topically to skin under an occlusive dressing. The most common use is in its application in paediatric practice to reduce the pain from venepuncture. It has also been used to provide analgesia at the donor site of skin grafts. A disadvantage is that it requires a waiting time of ½–1 h to produce its full analgesic effects.

Dosages

Fixed maximum doses of local anaesthetic agents can only be a guideline. Sensitivity to given doses will depend upon the size of the patient, site of injection, and presence of vasoconstrictor agents. The addition of vasoconstrictor drugs will generally reduce sensitivity to local anaesthetic agents in all sites of use except topically to the tracheo-bronchial tree where absorption is particularly rapid.

Effective concentrations and volumes of local anaesthetic agent vary widely with the differing techniques. When lignocaine is used, satisfactory infiltration analgesia can be obtained at low concentrations (0.5 per cent) whilst effective motor block during epidural anaesthesia will require higher concentrations (1.5-2 per cent).

Time of onset and duration of effect of commonly used local anaesthetic agents are listed in Table 13.2.

Table 13.2 Time course of actions of local anaesthetic agents and suggested maximum doses

Agent	Onset (min)	Duration (h)	Maximum dosage (mg/kg)
Lignocaine	10-15	1-3	3
Lignocaine + Adren	10-15	3-4	7
Prilocaine	10-15	1.5-2	5
Prilocaine + Adren	10-15	2-3	8
Bupivacaine 0.25%	15-30	3-5	2
Bupivacaine 0.5%	15-30	3-6	2
Bupivacaine + Adren	15-30	3-6	2

Absorption of the local anaesthetic agent from the site of injection into tissues and blood vessels is also dependent upon the lipid solubility of the individual agent. As local anaesthetic agents are relatively lipid soluble, diffusion across capillary endothelium will be rapid and systemic absorption rates will be dependent upon blood flow and binding to local tissues. The vascularity of the site of injection is therefore important; rapid and extensive absorption will take place from inflamed and highly vascular tissues. Vasoconstrictor drugs will reduce the vascular absorption of the local anaesthetic agents. In general, systemic absorption rate is related to the site of injection (see Table 13.3). Absorption decreases in the following order—*intercostal >caudal >epidural >brachial plexus >sciatic* and *femoral blocks*.

Vasoconstrictor agents such as adrenalin, at concentrations of 1:100 000–1:400 000, phenylephrine, felypressin, and octapressin are often used to reduce drug absorption and prolong the duration of anaesthetic effects. They produce little prolongation of action with the long-acting local anaesthetic agents such as bupivacaine.

Table 13.3 Absorption of local anaesthetic drugs and site of injection

Intercostal	Rapid
Caudal	↓
Epidural	↓
Brachial plexus	↓
Sciatic and femoral	Slow

TOXICITY OF LOCAL ANAESTHETICS

When administered in an appropriate dose and in a correct anatomical location, local anaesthetics are relatively free from toxic effects. However, local and systemic toxic effects may follow the administration of an excessive dose of local anaesthetic agent or following accidental intravascular or intrathecal injection.

Local effects

Local tissue toxicity

Nerve damage in experimental animals has been seen following excessive doses of local anaesthetic agents. In addition, preservative agents, notably sodium bisulphite, may be neurotoxic. Skeletal muscle changes have been observed with most of the local anaesthetic agents and the irritant properties of local anaesthetic agents may be responsible, although the changes have not correlated with clinically overt signs of local irritation. The damage is reversible and regeneration complete within two weeks.

These effects are mostly experimental and do not appear to cause problems in clinical practice.

Vascular damage

If vasoconstrictor drugs such as adrenalin are used, spasm of blood vessels may result. In areas of the body supplied by end-arteries (ear lobes, nose, digits, penis) this may result in necrosis.

Systemic effects

Cardiovascular system

Local anaesthetic agents, by virtue of their membrane-stabilizing properties, reduce cardiac irritability, and impulse conduction time is prolonged. All agents are negative inotropes and reduce myocardial contractility. These properties can produce direct impairment of cardiac function if large amounts are absorbed or after inadvertent intravenous injection.

Vasodilatation occurs as a result of direct relaxant effects on smooth muscle with some local anaesthetic agents. In addition, the reduced cardiac output, resulting from the direct cardiac depressant effects, and the hypotension result in tissue hypoxia and a metabolic acidosis. This further impairs myocardial function. Cardiovascular depression resulting from toxic effects of bupivacaine has proved refractory to resuscitation attempts. An adequate circulation must be established, to enable drug redistribution and metabolism of the drug in the liver, and thereby reduce toxic plasma-concentrations of bupivacaine. Prolonged cardiopulmonary resuscitation may be required and, on occasions, cardiopulmonary bypass has been instituted to support the cardiovascular system.

Central nervous system

Initially, central nervous system excitation is seen as a result of inhibition of cortical inhibitory synapses, and convulsions will occur. Larger doses will produce generalized central nervous system depression.

Symptoms of toxicity

At the onset of toxic effects, the patient may complain of a feeling of numbness, characteristically of tongue and lips, and general light-headedness. Tinnitus and visual disturbance are other frequent complaints that should alert one to the risk of systemic toxicity. These are summarized in Table 13.4.

Table 13.4   Signs of systemic toxicity of local anaesthetics

---

Tinnitus

Restlessness

Muscle twitching

Loss of consciousness

Generalized convulsions

Respiratory arrest

Hypotension

Asystole (bupivacaine may produce ventricular dysrhythmias)

Management of systemic toxicity

Drugs and equipment necessary for the management of systemic toxicity of local anaesthetic agents should be available wherever these drugs are used other than for skin infiltration and distal-limb nerve blocks, and the operator must be familiar with the treatment required.

Problems may arise as a result of the profound cardiovascular depression which occurs with hypotension and cardiac arrest. The depression of the central nervous system, leading to respiratory depression, hypoxia, and acidosis, may be the primary cause of the collapse, with the cardiovascular problems secondary events Resuscitation should be directed to improving both of these.

Minimum resuscitation equipment

1. Fully trained staff familiar with cardiopulmonary resuscitation at basic and advanced levels must be available.
2. Oxygen supply, masks, and a self-inflating bag to enable manual assistance of ventilation during resuscitation.

3. Suction apparatus. When consciousness is impaired or lost the patient is at risk of aspiration of gastric contents.

4. Tracheal intubation equipment will be necessary to facilitate tracheal intubation, both to protect the airway in the unconscious patient and for assistance of ventilation. Laryngoscopes and cuffed tracheal tubes of appropriate adult and paediatric sizes should be available.

5. Anticonvulsant drugs should be available—benzodiazepines, e.g. Diazemuls, or a barbiturate such as thiopentone. Suxamethonium, a short-acting, depolarizing muscle relaxant, may be used by an anaesthetist to facilitate intubation.

6. Sympathomimetic drugs to treat hypotension may be required. Ephedrine in 5 mg boluses, given intravenously, is effective.

7. Anti-arrhythmic drugs may be necessary. Bradycardia may be treated with intravenous atropine. Adrenalin will be required in cases of asystole. Other dysrhythmias may improve once hypoxia has been corrected and cardiac output has improved with the previous measures.

8. When performing major conduction-nerve blocks such as epidural or spinal blocks, a tilting bed, table, or trolley on which the patient may be rapidly placed in the head down (Trendelenberg) position is essential. This will increase venous return and, in patients with profound sympathetic blockade after spinal or epidural block, this will counteract the venous pooling in the lower limbs.

Reactions to vasoconstrictor drugs

Vasoconstrictor drugs are used in combination with local anaesthetic agents to retard drug absorption and reduce systemic drug toxicity. In addition, by maintaining effective tissue drug concentrations they prolong the duration of action of some local anaesthetic drugs. Reactions to the vasoconstrictor agent may be seen and are usually related to systemic absorption or intravenous injection. Symptoms include anxiety and palpitations; the patient will appear pale and develop a tachycardia, hypertension, and rapid respiratory rate. These effects are usually transient, the agents being rapidly metabolized.

Allergic reactions to local anaesthetic drugs

These are rare reactions, particularly with the amide group of drugs. When ester drugs such as procaine were commonly used, skin reactions resulting from handling were observed.

Treatment of allergic reactions include general supportive measures to ensure adequate oxygenation and specific therapies to minimize the immunological reactions. Hypotension should initially be managed with intravenous fluids and bronchospasm requires the administration of β_2-adrenoceptor stimulants, the drug of first choice being adrenalin. Steroids may be given intravenously and systemic antihistamines may be administered.

Applications of local analgesic techniques in acute pain

This section provides a brief review of some of the techniques available to relieve acute pain. Some techniques (indicated in the text by an asterisk *) are only suitable to be performed by persons trained in anaesthesia.

Topical

Local anaesthetic agents may be applied to mucous membranes to produce localized areas of analgesia. This may be particularly useful in painful lesions of the mouth and oropharynx. Suitable agents include lozenges of benzocaine or amethocaine. A topical, 0.5 per cent solution of amethocaine is available and provides useful anaesthesia of the cornea for procedures such as removal of foreign body or for analgesia after corneal abrasions.

Topical application of bupivacaine to the donor sites of skin grafts has also been found to provide good analgesia postoperatively. EMLA cream may also be useful in this situation.

Local infiltration

This method of producing local anaesthesia may be useful after trauma—for example, prior to suturing of simple wounds or for the infiltration of fracture sites prior to manipulation.

Local anaesthetic agents may be infiltrated into surgical wounds at the end of an operation to provide analgesia well into the postoperative period. This has been found to be particularly useful after procedures such as orchidopexy and herniotomy in children. Catheters inserted in surgical wounds at the time of operation have also been used to enable intermittent injections of local anaesthetic agents to be repeated in the postoperative period to provide prolonged analgesia. However, the analgesia produced is often patchy and concern that the presence of the catheter in the wound may increase the risk of postoperative wound infections has prevented its widespread acceptance.

Nerve blocks

Injection of local anaesthetic near the nerve or nerves supplying the painful area may be useful after traumatic injury and for postoperative pain. Some examples of those commonly used include ring block for digital nerves (p. 113), intercostal nerve blocks for pain relief after abdominal and thoracic surgical procedures (p. 114), and femoral nerve block for pain after a fractured femur (p. 117). Similarly, individual nerves at the wrist or ankle may be blocked to provide areas of analgesia.

The peripheral nerves to the upper limb are invested in a connective-tissue sheath and this anatomical arrangement has allowed the development of techniques that provide analgesia to the arm using blockade of the brachial plexus. Axillary*, supraclavicular*, and interscalene* approaches to the brachial plexus sheath have been described and used for anaesthesia for surgical procedures and for postoperative analgesia. Prolonged analgesia can be maintained if a small catheter is placed into the sheath and used to administer repeated doses of local anaesthetic agents to maintain the blockade. A useful adjunct to this block is the local sympathetic blockade also produced, which may be beneficial in improving peripheral blood flow to the damaged limb or after surgical procedures involving the vasculature of the upper limb.

Field block

This technique involves the injection of local anaesthetic agent so as to create a zone of analgesia around the site of the wound. It may involve both nerve block and skin-infiltration elements. This technique can be used to provide surgical anaesthesia for inguinal hernia repairs but may also be used for postoperative analgesia after such procedures.

Epidural* and spinal* local analgesic blocks
See Chapter 14.

Choice of local anaesthetic agent
Suitable local anaesthetic agents for the various techniques described are listed in Table 13.5.

Table 13.5   Choice of local anaesthetic agent

Procedure	Agent
Topical	
Bronchoscopy	Lignocaine 4%
ENT procedures	
Nasal operations	Cocaine
Oral	Benzocaine
Venepuncture	EMLA
Infiltration	
Wound	Lignocaine 0.5-1%
Fracture site	Bupivacaine 0.25%
	Prilocaine 0.5%
Nerve block	Lignocaine 1-2%
	Bupivacaine 0.25-0.5%
	Prilocaine 0.5-1%
Epidural	Lignocaine 1.5-2%
	with adrenalin
	Bupivacaine 0.25-0.5%
	(Ropivacaine 0.5-1%)
Spinal	Lignocaine 5%
	hyperbaric
	Bupivacaine 0.5%
	isobaric/hyperbaric

14 Local anaesthetic techniques—practical procedures

Some useful nerve blocks are described in this chapter. Not all of the techniques are suitable for readers of this book to perform but they are described in depth to encourage understanding amongst those who may not be familiar with the methods, but who may have to care for patients before or after nerve blocks. Other blocks described may well be suitable for house officers to perform. This book attempts to be complementary to more specialized instruction manuals and is not a substitute for adequate instruction in the practical points.

It is expected that before performing these nerve blocks, doctors will be proficient in resuscitation skills and that immediate access to resuscitation equipment, drugs, and assistance is available.

General contra-indications to local anaesthetic procedures

- Patient acceptance of any local anaesthetic technique is a prime consideration. Unwillingness to have any block performed should be accepted by the doctor and the patient should not be pressurized into agreeing to the procedure. Anxiety about the procedure and risks can usually be allayed with adequate information and sensitive reassurance.

- Sepsis at the proposed site of injection is a contraindication to all forms of local anaesthetic block. Spread of infection directly from the needle or intravascularly may result in abscess formation and significant morbidity. This is particularly important with techniques such as epidural or spinal blocks where the effects of abscesses may permanently damage spinal cord function.

- Central nervous system or spinal disorders are often considered to be contra-indications to epidural and spinal blocks. However, it is unlikely that these blocks affect the course of a chronic neurological disease such as multiple sclerosis.

- Patients receiving anticoagulant therapy—warfarin or subcutaneous heparin—will be at greater risk of haematoma formation whatever block is used and advice over the suitability of the technique should be sought. Epidural and spinal blocks are contra-indicated.

- Obesity and skeletal abnormalities may increase the difficulties associated with the performance of the block. Surface landmarks for deeper structures may be unreliable. Positioning the patient may also be difficult.

If difficulties are experienced in performing local analgesic techniques—do not persist—get help.

General principles of regional anaesthesia

1. Ask the patient about any previous exposure to local anaesthetic techniques—most often these are associated with dental procedures—and whether there were any complications of the procedure.

2. Examine the patient before performing a local anaesthetic block to ensure that you can identify the landmarks and there are no signs of sepsis at the proposed site of injection.

3. Explain the procedure to the patient, the expected effects, and the duration of the block. This is particularly important if temporary motor paralysis may occur with the nerve block or if prolonged sensory blockade may be experienced by the patient.

4. Note any concomitant medication that may influence your choice of technique.

5. All drugs and equipment required for performing the block should be assembled and checked.

6. Check that resuscitation equipment and drugs are available.

7. Before any block where potentially toxic doses of local anaesthetic agents may be administered or physiological effects such as hypotension resulting from the block itself may be expected, intravenous access should be obtained and secured. This enables rapid treatment of any adverse effects from the block or from systemic toxicity of the local anaesthetic agent used.

8. Before injecting any local anaesthetic always aspirate the syringe first. If blood is obtained do not inject the local anaesthetic. Even small amounts given intravenously can produce serious toxicity.

9. The patient should be monitored during the procedure. When epidural and spinal blocks are being performed this may include an ECG and automatic blood-pressure recordings to detect hypotension occurring as a result of the sympathetic blockade produced by the technique.

10. The patient should be positioned appropriately for the particular technique to be performed.

11. An aseptic technique must be used for all blocks. The person performing the nerve block should be scrubbed and wear sterile gloves. Gowns may be worn, in addition, when performing epidural and spinal blocks. The skin area where the nerve block will be performed should be cleaned with antiseptic solutions of iodine, chlorhexidine, or alcohol and covered with sterile drapes.

12. Perform the block. Communication should be maintained with the patient throughout the procedure. If paraesthesiae are to be elicited to identify the position of the needle the patient should be warned to expect 'pins and needles' and their distribution. This should prevent inadvertent movement in response to these sensations which will reduce the risk of needle displacement. If any untoward effects such as tinnitus, dizziness, or pain with injection of the local anaesthetic are felt the patient should be asked to report them.

13. The early signs of systemic toxicity (p. 103) should be sought during injection of the local anaesthetic solution. If they occur—stop the injection and begin appropriate treatment.

14. Observe the patient. Remember that no analgesic technique is 100 per cent effective all the time. Further analgesia or modification to the technique may be required.

PRACTICAL PROCEDURES

Wound infiltration/instillation

Indications

- Postoperative analgesia: herniotomy, orchidopexy in children, herniorrhaphy in adults.
- Prior to suture: skin lacerations, episiotomy repairs.

Technique

Wound instillation is commonly performed at the end of the operative procedure and may be performed at the closure of the wound at both deep and superficial levels. A suitable agent would be bupivacaine 0.25 per cent at doses of 0.5 ml/kg in children. Infiltration of local anaesthetic subcutaneously along the wound edges may be performed for anaesthesia prior to suturing of simple wounds or lacerations. It will provide analgesia after surgery.

Digital nerve block

Indications

- Trauma: prior to suture of lacerations to fingers/toes.
- Surgery: local anaesthesia for surgical operations to fingers/toes.

Anatomy

The major digital nerves run on the ventrolateral aspects of the fingers/toes and are accompanied by the digital vessels. They give off articular branches and also a dorsal branch to supply the nail bed. In the hand these main nerves originate from the median and ulnar nerves; further small dorsal digital nerves originating from the radial nerve supply the dorsum of the fingers.

Technique

The digital nerves may be blocked at each side of the digit at the proximal phalanx. Injections of 1–2 ml of 2 per cent lignocaine should be made from the dorsal aspect, on each side, into the finger through skin weals using a 23 or 25 G needle. A further 1–2 ml may be infiltrated along the dorsal aspect of the digit between the two injection sites to ensure blockade of the dorsal branches. Analgesia may take 10–15 min to develop. This technique is suitable for minor surgical procedures such as toe-nail removal and suturing of lacerations.

Intercostal nerve block

Indications

- Trauma—rib fractures.
- Surgery—thoracic/abdominal.

Anatomy

The intercostal nerves run segmentally under the lower border of the respective ribs, between the external and internal intercostal muscles. They supply the intercostal muscles, transversus thoracis, and the abdominal muscles. They are sensory for the chest wall and abdomen. For analgesia of the abdominal wall, blockade of T5–T12 is required.

Technique

Intercostal nerve block is best performed in the mid-axillary line with the patient supine. The arm should be fully abducted and held anteriorly, elevating the scapula and allowing access to the intercostal nerves from the fourth nerve downwards. The caudad margin of the rib should be palpated between the finger and thumb of the left hand and the overlying skin fixed. A 21 or 23 G needle attached to the syringe containing the local anaesthetic solution is inserted towards the rib aiming to make contact with the rib just above the caudad edge. Once this contact has been made the needle should be angulated in a caudad direction and gradually 'walked off the rib' to pass just under the caudad border of the rib. The needle should be advanced approximately 2–3 mm from the surface of the rib. Careful aspiration of the syringe at this time is essential. If blood is obtained (indicating intravascular placement of the needle) or air (indicating pleural penetration) the needle should be withdrawn. Should no air or blood be obtained at aspiration then 2.5 ml of bupivacaine 0.5 per cent should be injected at each intercostal space to be blocked. As the needle is withdrawn, a further 0.5 ml of local anaesthetic can be injected to anaesthetize the site of entry. This will ensure that when blocks need to be repeated less discomfort will be experienced.

Bupivacaine is the local anaesthetic of choice providing prolonged analgesia—up to 12 h.

For mid-line abdominal wounds, complete analgesia following intercostal nerve blockade will require bilateral blocks.

Analgesia in the region of the xiphisternum will require blockade of the sixth to eighth intercostal nerves. To reach the umbilicus, blockade will need to extend to the tenth intercostal nerve (Fig. 14.1).

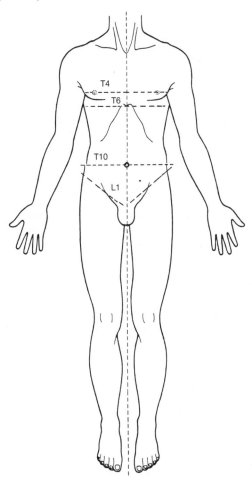

Fig. 14.1 Landmarks for levels of analgesia after intercostal nerve blockade.

Alternatively the intercostal nerves may be blocked posteriorly at the angle of the ribs. This is performed with the patient in a lateral position and the injection points are lateral to the erector spinae muscles, approximately 8 cm from the mid-line. Again the procedure should be to advance the needle until it slips under the caudad border of the rib, where 2–3 ml of bupivacaine should be injected after careful aspiration for blood and air. The patient's arms may need to be elevated across the chest to allow access to the sixth and seventh intercostal nerves by elevating the scapula. Bilateral blocks will require the patient to be turned to allow access to the opposite side.

Complications

The most important complication is the development of a pneumothorax resulting from lung puncture. Usually this is minor and will resolve spontaneously. Occasionally a tension pneumothorax may be produced and will require immediate insertion of an underwater-seal chest drain. If air is aspirated at any time during the performance of the blocks, an erect chest X-ray should be performed to detect the presence of a pneumothorax.

Care should be taken not to exceed the maximum doses of local anaesthetic when multiple blocks are to be performed. Local anaesthetic is absorbed rapidly following intercostal nerve block because of the high vascularity of this region. Preparations containing adrenalin may be used to reduce absorption, and careful aspiration should be performed with each injection to prevent intravascular administration and systemic local anaesthetic toxicity.

Interpleural injection of local anaesthetic

The technique of interpleural local anaesthetic injection has provided good analgesia for patients who have undergone surgery through a subcostal incision. Local anaesthetic injected into the pleural space has been shown, using radio-opaque contrast, to spread from the diaphragm to the apex of the lung along the dorsal aspect of the pleural space. Analgesic effects may result from diffusion of the local anaesthetic through the dorsal subpleural space and blocking the intercostal nerves.

Indications
- Postoperative analgesia for surgery via a subcostal incision; for example, cholecystectomy.
- Analgesia following rib fractures.

Technique
The patient is placed in the left lateral position (for right-sided blocks) and the seventh intercostal space identified. The skin should be infiltrated with local anaesthetic and then a 16 G Tuohy needle introduced through the skin in the mid-axillary line. A glass syringe, partially full of air, is attached to the needle to detect loss of resistance as the pleural space is entered, at which time the plunger of the syringe should be sucked in. The syringe is then removed and an epidural catheter can be passed through the Tuohy needle leaving approximately 5 cm in the space. A microbiological filter is attached to the end of the catheter, which enables repeated injections to be given. The dose required to provide analgesia in adults is 20 ml of bupivacaine 0.5 per cent. Repeated injections may be required every 4–6 h. Catheters may be left in place for up to 72 h.

In patients who have suffered chest trauma where there is already a chest drain *in situ* this may also be used as a portal of entry. The local anaesthetic may be instilled through the chest drain, which should be clamped (though only in patients with no air leak) for a short period (20–30 min) to allow time for the local anaesthetic to be effective.

Complications
There is a risk of pneumothorax from the procedure but this rarely requires insertion of a chest drain.

Incorrect positioning of the catheter can lead to inadequate analgesia.

Femoral nerve block

Indications
- Fractured shaft of femur.
- Surgery/trauma to thigh and knee.
- Surgery/trauma to lower leg—in combination with sciatic nerve blockade.

Femoral nerve block is ideally suited for the immediate care of patients with fractures of the shaft of the femur. Good analgesia is produced within 10 min and enables the patient to be examined and X-rayed with minimal discomfort. Good motor blockade from bupivacaine also reduces painful muscle spasm that is commonly associated with the fracture.

Anatomy

The femoral nerve runs from the lumbar plexus between the psoas and iliac muscles and enters the thigh by passing deep to the inguinal ligament. It innervates the skin of the anterior thigh and medial side of the calf down to the medial malleolus. It also has branches to the quadriceps muscles, sartorius muscle, and supplies the knee joint.

Technique

The femoral nerve is accessible, in its neurovascular sheath, just below the inguinal ligament.

Standing on the opposite side to that on which the block is to be performed, the pulsation of the femoral artery should be palpated just below the inguinal ligament. The injection site is immediately lateral to the femoral artery and the needle should be directed cephalad. Paraesthesiae may be obtained in the conscious patient indicating the correct position of the needle. In unconscious patients the injection should be made in a fan-like manner to a depth of 3–5 cm, aspirating at each injection. If firm digital pressure is maintained distal to the injection site, local anaesthetic in the neurovascular sheath will be directed cephalad, blocking the obturator nerve and the lateral femoral cutaneous nerve of the thigh—the so-called '3-in-1' block.

Bupivacaine 0.25 or 0.5 per cent are the local anaesthetic agents of choice for this block. In adults, volumes of 20 ml should be used. When the 3-in-1 block is performed, 30 ml of local anaesthetic solution may be required.

Epidural and spinal blockade

Spinal anaesthesia

The earliest reported use of spinal anaesthesia in man was by Auguste Bier, in 1898, who injected cocaine intrathecally. The technique was further developed and used widely with newer local anaesthetic agents. Fears of neurological complications following spinal anaesthesia led to a decline in its popularity in the UK in the 1950s. These fears have since been felt to be unjustified and spinal anaesthesia is now recognized as a safe and effective technique. It is principally used to provide anaesthesia for surgical procedures below the umbilicus—particularly for orthopaedic and urological operations. With most of the currently available local anaesthetic agents for spinal use, the blockade produced is of relatively short duration and provides little postoperative analgesia. Techniques using the insertion of catheters into the subarachnoid space have been used to provide analgesia by continuous administration of local anaesthetic providing a prolonged block. Since the catheters must be inserted intrathecally and may provide a portal of entry for bacteria this technique has not been widely used.

The effects of local anaesthetic agents on nerve conduction are seen first on the smaller diameter fibres—pre-ganglionic sympathetic fibres being the most easily blocked. Sensory modalities are blocked in the order of increasing fibre diameter—temperature, pain, touch, and pressure. The final level of blockade is of the motor and proprioception pathways.

The extent of blockade achieved after subarachnoid injection of local anaesthetic agents is variable. This may result from a number of factors.

- Patient position—during and after injection of the local anaesthetic solution. Sitting a patient up may produce a more profound block in the sacral roots.

- Specific gravity of local anaesthetic solutions—spread of the local anaesthetic agents within the CSF is altered if hyperbaric, isobaric, or hypobaric solutions are used. Hyperbaric solutions will tend to produce more profound effects in the more dependent regions, in contrast to hypobaric solutions where the effects will be more concentrated in the uppermost regions.

- Site of injection—blockade will be produced more rapidly and more extensively in regions close to the site of injection. In addition, the curvatures of the spine in the thoracic and lumbar regions will tend to limit the spread of solution injected at distal sites and therefore limit the extent of the block.

- Volume and dose of drug injected—the extent of blockade will be greater with both larger doses of drug and greater volumes injected into the CSF.

Suitable agents are listed in Table 14.1.

Table 14.1   Local anaesthetic agents for spinal blocks

Agent	Dose (mg)		Duration (min)
	T10	T4	
Lignocaine 5%	30-50	75-100	45-60
Bupivacaine 0.5% isobaric	10-15	15-20	150-200
Bupivacaine 0.5% hyperbaric	15	20	90-110

Local anaesthetic agents for spinal use have been prepared in solutions of differing specific gravity in attempts to alter the spread of local anaesthetic. Solutions are available as isobaric, hypobaric, and hyperbaric when compared with CSF. By combining the particular preparation with posture it is possible to influence the spread of local anaesthetic blockade. Examples include the following.

Saddle block   Typically this utilizes a hyperbaric local anaesthetic solution injected in a low lumbar interspace with the patient in a sitting position. This leads to the development of a block principally in the sacral region, suitable for operations in the region of distribution of the sacral nerve roots such as haemorrhoidectomy.

Unilateral block   This technique again uses hyperbaric anaesthetic solution. A predominantly unilateral block is obtained by injection with the patient lying on the side that is to be anaesthetized. Alternatively if a hypobaric solution is used the principal effects of the block would be on the uppermost side.

Epidural analgesia
The epidural space is a loose connective-tissue filled space between the outer layer of the spinal dura and the vertebral canal. It

extends from the foramen magnum to the sacral hiatus. The contents of the space include the dural sac and spinal nerve roots, the epidural venous plexus, and the spinal arteries, lymphatic vessels, and fat. The average width of the space is 0.5 cm although it is at its largest in the lumbar region.

When a solution of local anaesthetic agent is injected into the epidural space it may exert its effects either on nerve roots in the epidural or paravertebral spaces or intradurally after diffusion through the dura into the subarachnoid space. An analgesic solution injected into the epidural space may spread caudally and cephalad, extending the region of blockade. Many factors may influence the extent of spread of the local anaesthetic agent in the epidural space including the following.

- Amount of local anaesthetic agent—overall effects of the block are related to the total dose of drug administered. In children, doses may be calculated on a mg/kg basis and when the caudal route is used as access to the epidural space in children these doses can produce predictable blockade.

- Volume of local anaesthetic solution—although the total dose of drug administered is of major importance the concentration, and thereby the volume, in which this is administered may also influence the extent of the block although this is often unpredictable. In general the extent of the block may be greater if the same mass of drug is injected in a greater volume of solution.

- Patient age—the elderly require less drug than the young to produce the same extent of blockade.

- Pregnancy—less drug is required to produce a similar extent of blockade in pregnant patients compared with the non-pregnant state.

- Site of injection—spread of local anaesthetic produces a more extensive blockade after injection in the thoracic region compared with the lumbar region.

- Local anaesthetic agent used—different local anaesthetic agents can produce different profiles in extent and nature of blockade. Etidocaine produces a more profound motor block than bupivacaine.

- Positioning of the patient—during and immediately after the injection in a similar manner to the effects occurring after spinal anaesthesia.

The extent of blockade required for epidural and spinal techniques for surgical procedures is given in Table 14.2.

Table 14.2   Levels of spinal and epidural anaesthesia required for surgical procedures

Level	Surgical procedure
T4-5 (nipple)	Upper abdominal surgery
T6-8 (xiphoid)	Intestinal surgery, gynaecological surgery, ureter, and renal pelvic surgery
T10 (umbilicus)	Transurethral resection, obstetric vaginal delivery, hip surgery
L1 (inguinal ligament)	Thigh surgery, lower limb amputations, etc.
L2-3 (knee and below)	Foot surgery
S2-5 (perineal)	Perineal surgery, haemorrhoidectomy, etc.

Epidural blockade

Indications

- Lumbar: lower abdominal / lower limb surgery; obstetric analgesia / anaesthesia.
- Thoracic: upper abdominal surgery / thoracic surgery; chest trauma.

Contra-indications

(1) Bleeding tendency;
(2) local sepsis at site of epidural;
(3) hypotension;
(4) raised intracranial pressure;
(5) acute neurological conditions;
(6) patient refusal.

Relative contra-indications:

(1) Difficult anatomy.

Anatomy
See p. 121.

Technique

See the suggested additional reading for the details of this procedure.

The development of the block can be monitored using both sensory loss (to cold or pinprick) and motor paralysis (inability to raise the legs).

Management of an epidural block

For prolonged analgesia a catheter is inserted into the epidural space allowing repeated administration of local anaesthetic.

Bupivacaine is the most commonly used local anaesthetic for epidural blockade. Incremental doses of 5–10 ml of 0.25 or 0.5 per cent solutions may be given intermittently to maintain an appropriate level of analgesia. Alternatively a continuous infusion of local anaesthetic solution may be maintained.

Patient monitoring
Intravenous access must be maintained in all patients until the effects of the block have worn off.

Regular monitoring of the patient is important to ensure adequate levels of analgesia and, when using infusion techniques, that these levels do not extend progressively higher.

Repeated checks of blood pressure are mandatory and must be performed at frequent intervals after each top-up bolus dose to detect any hypotension developing from sympathetic effects.

Complications
1. Intravascular administration of local anaesthetic. This will result in the signs and symptoms of systemic local anaesthetic toxicity (p. 104).

2. Hypotension may occur as a result of the blockade of the sympathetic fibres producing vasodilatation in the area of the block. This should be treated with ephedrine (5 mg boluses IV) and intravenous volume expansion (1–2 l of 0.9% Saline). Hypotension is accentuated in the pregnant patient particularly when lying supine. This results from the aorto-caval compression from the gravid uterus. Hypotensive pregnant patients should therefore always be turned on to their sides and intravenous fluids and vasopressors administered if this manoeuvre does not improve the blood pressure.

3. Subarachnoid administration of local anaesthetic will result in the extension of the block to high levels, usually following a bolus (top-up) dose. It may occur through inadvertent, unrecognized dural puncture at the time of performing the block, or some time after if the catheter has migrated through the dura. The signs are of a rapidly developing, extensive sensory and motor blockade. Respiratory difficulties may occur with blocks which progress above the level of T4 although diaphragmatic function should be preserved unless the block extends higher than C3–5. Tingling and numbness may be experienced in the hands as the block progresses to higher thoracic and cervical dermatomes.

Should this occur it is important to reassure the patient and explain what is occurring. Oxygen should be administered and respiratory support (tracheal intubation, and assisted ventilation) may be required.

High blocks will usually be associated with profound hypotension as the sympathetic nerves will also be affected. Administer intravenous colloids (1–2 l of a gelatin solution) and vasopressors (ephedrine in 5 mg increments given IV). Bardycardia resulting from blockade of the cardiac sympathetics can be treated with atropine (1–2 mg IV).

Should this situation occur it is important to remember to sedate the patient once the airway is secure, ventilation is supported, and an adequate blood pressure established.

4. Headaches (see p. 127).

Epidural catheters
These are fine-gauge catheters that can be placed in the epidural space and through which intermittent injections or infusions of

local anaesthetic agents can be given. They can have a single end-hole or multiple holes with a rounded end. There is debate as to how long a catheter may be left in the epidural space. Ideally catheters should be removed after 72 h although they may be left up to a week without complications. There have been reports of catheters being in place for up to two weeks without difficulties. It is important that strict adherence to asepsis occurs while siting the epidural. The use of microbiological filters attached to the catheter also reduces the incidence of catheter infections.

Catheters should be removed with gentle traction at the skin entry site. Once removed the catheter must be checked to ensure that it has all been removed. If, during removal, resistance is felt, gentle continuous traction with the spine flexed may help. Generally only 2–4 cm of catheter are left in the epidural space and the risk of knots in the catheter is low. If continued difficulty is experienced, the catheter may have caught around a nerve root in which case the patient will complain of pain when traction is applied to the catheter. Should this occur the catheter should be left in position and radiographs taken with contrast injected through the catheter to localize its position. If it is located in the vicinity of a nerve root, removal by formal laminectomy may be necessary.

If on removal the catheter is found to have fractured, leaving small amounts in the epidural space, this should be recorded in the patient's notes and the patient informed. Small fragments are unlikely to require surgical removal and may prove difficult to locate if laminectomy is performed.

Epidural top-up procedures

These are suggested instructions that may be left for nurses when epidurals are managed by them. Epidurals using local anaesthetic agents should not be routinely managed on general wards but only in high dependency or intensive care units because of the hazards involved.

1. Check prescription and volume and concentration of local anaesthetic.
2. Check the level of sensory block still present and if still high while the patient is in pain call the doctor/anaesthetist for advice.

3. Check that the intravenous infusion is running.
4. Aspirate the epidural catheter, looking for evidence of blood or free flow of cerebrospinal fluid.
5. Give 3 ml of the local anaesthetic as a small test-dose and monitor for any unwanted effects.
6. Give the remainder of the dose slowly if no complications have occurred after the initial dose.
7. Ensure appropriate monitoring of the patient—blood pressure, level of block, at 5 min intervals for 30 min after each top-up.
8. Inform the doctor or anaesthetist if the systolic blood pressure decreases below 90 mm Hg.

Caudal approach to the epidural space

The epidural space may also be approached through the sacral hiatus. This is a particularly useful route for producing blockade of the lower sacral nerve roots. It is used for perineal surgery or for postoperative analgesia following procedures such as haemorrhoidectomy. It is widely used in children, when the sacral hiatus is easily accessible and can be used to provide analgesia following circumcision, orchidopexy, and herniotomy.

The place of epidural analgesia

Although it is time consuming and requires expertise to site the epidural catheter it must be appreciated that this is only the beginning of the extra work and patient care that providing epidural analgesia will require. It has become an accepted technique in the obstetric unit and the extra workload and demands on staff have been accommodated from within the midwifery and anaesthetic services. For the patient with acute pain on a medical or surgical ward the complexities may limit its use to those in severe pain or those in whom parenteral opioids would be a disadvantage. If adequate and safe care for the patient cannot be provided on a general ward then the risks of the technique may outweigh the benefits from improved analgesia. The technique will therefore be generally confined to those patients receiving intensive nursing care. It is hoped that eventually, postoperative wards or recovery units will be available, allowing the management of patients with epidural catheters for analgesia.

Opioids versus local anaesthetics

With local anaesthetics, the epidural catheter must be sited in close proximity to the area in which the blockade is required. The local anaesthetic may be administered either by continuous infusion with a risk of increasing levels of block or by repeated top-up doses with risks of episodes of hypotension or acute toxicity. Experienced staff are required to carry out repeat injections and to deal with the adverse effects.

Opioid drugs will provide a much longer duration of analgesia and without the attendant risks of hypotension. Catheters sited in the lumbar region, technically easier than siting in the thoracic region, can be used with opioid drugs, as spread of the drug from the site of the injection is rapid. There is no motor blockade and other sensory modalities are unaffected with the opioids. However, all drugs have potential for producing delayed respiratory depression.

POST-LUMBAR-PUNCTURE HEADACHE

Headache can be one of the most disabling complications after spinal blocks or epidural blockade where the dura has been breached deliberately or inadvertently. It usually occurs within one to four days of the procedure and is made worse by the upright position and by coughing and straining. The pain is usually located in the occipital region and may be associated with neck stiffness. The headache is believed to be related to the leak of cerebrospinal fluid through the dura and efforts to reduce the incidence of headache have centred around the use of smaller needles to reduce the dural puncture size (see Table 14.3).

Table 14.3

Incidence of headache (per cent)	Needle size
75	17 G
12	22 G
1-3	25/26 G

The headache may last for 1–2 weeks but there are occasional reports of headache persisting for months.

Management of post-lumbar-puncture headache

1. Give adequate, regular simple analgesics, such as paracetamol or other NSAIDs.
2. Maintain hydration—regular oral fluids, or if the patient is unable to take oral fluids, then the intravenous route should be used.
3. Avoidance of coughing and straining—stool-softening agents or laxatives such as lactulose may be useful.
4. Bed rest is usually necessary simply because the headache is worse when the patient is upright.
5. The anaesthetist responsible for performing the block should be informed. He or she will then be able to reassure the patient and monitor the response to the simple measures described above. If, despite these measures, the headache persists the anaesthetist may then inject 10–20 ml of autologous blood into the epidural space to stop the CSF leak ('epidural blood patch'). This technique is usually rapidly effective.

Alternative therapies described to alleviate the headache include the use of large doses of caffeine, either orally or intravenously. Although this has been successful in some cases it may provide only temporary improvement.

15 Inhalational techniques and alternative therapies

Probably the earliest form of inhalational analgesia was the smoking of opium, addicts absorbing the inhaled vaporized drug. Most recently the inhalational route has been restricted to the use of a 50 per cent nitrous oxide/oxygen mixture—*Entonox*. Trichloroethylene and methoxyflurane, both anaesthetic vapours, have been used in low inhaled concentrations for analgesia. Methoxyflurane has been withdrawn from use due to its nephrotoxic effects, and trichloroethylene is about to be withdrawn.

When the inhalational route is used the blood concentration of the agent reaches an equilibrium at a rate dependent upon the alveolar minute ventilation and the solubility of the agent in the blood. Insoluble agents such as nitrous oxide reach analgesic blood concentrations more rapidly than more soluble agents such as methoxyflurane and trichloroethylene. Similarly once inhalation of the agent has been discontinued the analgesic effects of the insoluble agents wear off more rapidly.

Entonox

Nitrous oxide is an anaesthetic gas with potent analgesic effects. However, individual variation is wide with some patients showing marked sedation at inspired concentrations of 30–50 per cent. It is commonly used in general anaesthetic techniques but not as the sole anaesthetic agent.

When used as an analgesic agent it is administered premixed as Entonox, 50 per cent nitrous oxide in 50 per cent oxygen. It is distributed in cylinders that are coloured blue with white quartered collars. In some hospitals there may be pipeline supplies of Entonox to areas such as obstetric units where it is a valuable and frequently used analgesic agent. It is administered through a two-stage valve, the first stage a valve to reduce the pressure from the cylinder and then the second a patient-demand valve which opens as a result of the negative pressure generated by inspiration allowing inhalation on demand. A high flow rate must be supplied to match the peak inspiratory flow particularly in women in labour. Little inspiratory effort is required to trigger the valve and produce a high flow rate. The patient may either inhale through a mask or with a mouthpiece.

Nitrous oxide has a rapid onset and offset of analgesia and therefore finds a major use in situations where the pain is intermittent, exemplified by the painful contractions of labour or for postoperative patients when physiotherapy, removal of drains, or changes of dressings provoke pain of short duration. Typically analgesic effects are seen after approximately five breaths of Entonox. Patients should be instructed to inhale the Entonox for a short period of time, approximately 30 s, before the painful procedure such as the removal of drains is performed. Once the procedure is complete the inhalation can be discontinued. The technique thus requires patient co-operation, especially if analgesia needs to be maintained over a longer period of time.

Nitrous oxide is unsuitable for prolonged use due to its toxic effects, notably bone marrow depression, and also from the risks of environmental exposure to members of staff.

Entonox is a dry gas, and prolonged administration can be associated with discomfort due to drying of the mouth and upper airways.

The Entonox mask should be held over the face by the patients themselves. This is a safety feature of this method of administration; should the patient become excessively sedated the mask will fall away from the face. In such an event the patient will then breathe room air and rapidly awaken.

Contraindications to the use of Entonox
- Nitrous oxide will equilibrate with spaces containing air and replace the nitrogen. This results in an expansion of air spaces as the nitrous oxide diffuses into these spaces much more rapidly than the nitrogen diffuses out. This is important in patients with a pneumothorax, when expansion of the pneumothorax may occur and require urgent drainage. Air in other cavities such as the sinuses, middle ear, and also in the gut may also expand. Patients with intracranial air following trauma will also be at risk of increasing intracranial pressure with expansion of the air space.

- Sedation can occur with 50 per cent nitrous oxide and care must be taken in patients with depressed levels of consciousness following trauma.

Advantages
- Rapid onset and offset of analgesic effects.
- Useful for short procedures.
- Administration on demand.
- Patient control.
- Minimal cardiovascular depression.

Disadvantages
- Short duration of analgesic effects.
- Continuous inhalation requires effort and co-operation.
- Prolonged inhalation will produce drying of secretions and discomfort.
- Bulky nature of the equipment required for Entonox inhalation limits patient mobility.

ALTERNATIVE THERAPIES FOR PAIN CONTROL

Transcutaneous nerve stimulation

The application of transcutaneous electrical nerve stimulation (TENS) in the management of pain largely stems from the 'gate' theory described in Chapter 2. This theory suggests that if sensory input from large myelinated fibres is stimulated, this would close the gate to painful impulses transmitted by small C fibres. Clinical and experimental pain have both been shown to be reduced by electrical stimulation of peripheral nerves. TENS has been used for postoperative pain following thoracotomy, for analgesia after rib fractures, for acute low back pain, and is now widely used to provide analgesia during the first stage of labour.

The equipment consists of a pulse generator, an amplifier, and electrodes. The electrodes should be carefully applied, using electrode gel to reduce the impedance of the skin, to a site over peripheral nerves supplying the painful area. The frequency and intensity of the stimulus can be adjusted to the individual patient's requirements. Patients may control the equipment themselves after suitable training and familiarization with the equipment enabling maximum benefit to be obtained. Preoperative preparation and explanation in antenatal clinics in preparation for labour may be especially helpful.

Although controlled studies of its efficacy in acute pain vary widely in their results there may be a benefit in reducing opioid requirements and improving pulmonary function.

TENS is cheap, and appears to have few adverse effects. Both analgesia and adverse effects will diminish rapidly when the machine is disconnected.

Acupuncture

Traditional acupuncture is associated with the Chinese and has been practised for over 2000 years. The theory behind the insertion of needles at specific acupuncture points is that meridian lines were believed to exist in the body and that imbalance in the body would be expressed as pain. Specific sites along these meridians are related to different organs and regions of the body and appropriate points may be stimulated to relieve pain.

Acupuncture points are stimulated by the insertion of small solid needles into the appropriate location. The needle should be inserted deep into the muscle and a characteristic sensation often described as a tingling or numbness is felt by the patient. Modern techniques include electrical stimulation of the acupuncture needle using a pulse generator.

Acupuncture analgesia may partly be explained by the gate theory but it is also known to release endogenous opioid peptides and it can be reversed with the opioid antagonist naloxone.

16 Antiemetic drugs

Nausea and vomiting are frequent and distressing complications after surgery. In some patients they will occur after a minor body-surface operation associated with a brief general anaesthetic without opioids being used. In other patients their frequency, duration, and severity appear to be related to the magnitude of the procedure, type of anaesthesia, and consequent method of analgesia. Nausea and vomiting are particularly common after gastrointestinal surgery, as a result of postoperative gastrointestinal dysfunction. It may also be caused as an unwanted effect of the drugs that are used to control the pain. Some patients are particularly prone to vomiting and suitable reassurance and support may be important in these patients. Vomiting occurs more often in females than males and is more common in the young than in the elderly.

Vomiting is a reflex response which is controlled and co-ordinated by the brain-stem vomiting centre. This receives input from the medullary chemoreceptor trigger zone, from the vestibular centres, cerebellar nuclei, and cerebral cortex (Fig. 16.1).

Afferent pathways from the cerebellar and vestibular centres are susceptible to antagonism by centrally acting anticholinergic drugs, which are useful in treating motion sickness. Dopamine is a facilitatory neurotransmitter in the chemoreceptor trigger zone, receptors being principally of the D_2 type. Dopamine antagonist drugs will have antiemetic properties from action at this site. There is also evidence that dopamine may have peripheral effects on gastrointestinal mechanisms concerned with nausea and vomiting.

Before using pharmacological agents to relieve distress, other remediable causes should be sought. Starvation may be a cause of nausea and vomiting and early postoperative fluids may be therapeutic. Gastric distension resulting from ileus or from air swallowing may cause nausea and vomiting and this can be improved by the insertion of a nasogastric tube for drainage.

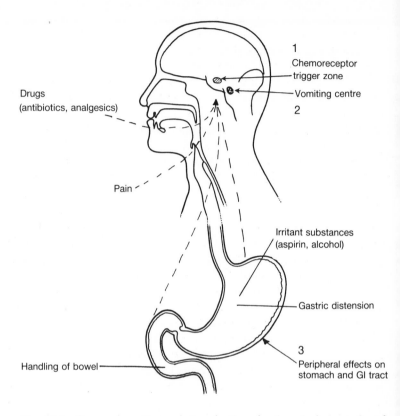

Fig. 16.1   Causes of vomiting and sites of action of antiemetic drugs. 1, 2, and
3 show the sites of action of antiemetic drugs.

Once remediable causes have been excluded, parenteral antiemetic therapy may be necessary to relieve distress. Oral administration may be used for prophylactic antiemetic therapy but
once vomiting is established this route is ineffective. Alternatively
many antiemetic drugs are available in suppository preparations
for rectal administration.

USEFUL ANTIEMETIC DRUGS

Phenothiazine derivatives
These drugs have antiemetic effects which result from their direct
actions on the chemoreceptor trigger zone. They are all dopamine

antagonists. These agents are the usual drugs for the first-line treatment of opioid-induced nausea and vomiting.

Complications of these drugs include acute dystonia typified by the occulo-gyric crisis, a distressing combination of involuntary muscular movements and spasm principally involving muscles of the face, head, and neck. This complication should be treated with intravenous *procyclidine* 5 mg, repeated if necessary after 30 min. The reversal of symptoms should occur within 5 min of injection.

Extrapyramidal effects are more common in children and the elderly and these drugs should be used with caution in these patient groups.

Chlorpromazine

Administered by injection, orally, or rectally this will reduce vomiting. Complications include hypotension, which results from its α-adrenoceptor blocking action and may be particularly marked in the hypovolaemic patient.

Adult doses: 25–50 mg IM, 3–4 hourly;
                10–25 mg oral, 4–6 hourly;
                100 mg suppository, 6–8 hourly.

Prochlorperazine

This drug is used for severe nausea and vomiting and is useful for treatment of symptoms of vertigo and labyrinthine disorders.

Adult doses: 12.5 mg IM, 6 hourly;
                5–10 mg oral, 8 hourly;
                25 mg suppository, 6 hourly.

Perphenazine

A useful drug for severe vomiting this agent is less sedative than chlorpromazine. Extrapyramidal symptoms are more common and the British National Formulary (BNF) suggests it should not be used in children.

Adult doses: 5–10 mg IM, 6 hourly (max. 15 mg in 24 h);
                2–4 mg oral, 8 hourly.

Thiethylperazine

This drug has actions at both the chemoreceptor trigger zone and the vomiting centre. Its duration of action is 6 h and hypotension, sedation, and extrapyramidal side-effects occur less often than with other phenothiazines.

Adult doses: 6.5 mg IM;
10 mg oral, 8–12 hourly;
6.5 mg suppository, 12 hourly.

Young adults are particularly susceptible to the extrapyramidal effects and the BNF again advises that this drug should not be used in children under 15 years of age.

Antihistamine drugs

These drugs act on the vomiting centre. They tend to be more sedative than other agents. There are no major advantages in antiemetic effect of one antihistamine over another but the drugs do differ markedly in the degree of sedation that occurs with different agents.

Cyclizine

In addition to its antihistamine effects this agent also has anticholinergic properties, which can produce unwanted effects of dry mouth and blurring of vision.

Adult doses: 50 mg IV, 8 hourly;
50 mg IM, 8 hourly;
50 mg oral, 8 hourly.

Paediatrics: 1–10 years, 25 mg oral, 8 hourly;
>10 years, 50 mg IM, 8 hourly.

Promethazine

This drug is generally more sedative than cyclizine. It is widely used in obstetric practice or as a premedicant drug.

Adult doses: 25 mg IV;
25–50 mg IM, 8 hourly;
25–50 mg oral—daily in divided doses.

Paediatrics: 1–5 years, 5 mg oral, 8 hourly;
     5–10 years, 10 mg oral, 8 hourly;
     6–12 years, 6.25–12.5 mg IM.

Anticholinergic drugs

Antiemetic actions may be peripheral, as a result of antagonism of acetylcholine effects on the gastrointestinal tract, and central nervous system effects.

Hyoscine (Scopolamine)

This agent is the most widely used mostly for the protective effect against nausea and vomiting induced by motion and labyrinthine disorders. Its central effects result in pronounced sedation particularly in the elderly. Most recently a transdermal preparation has been marketed for the control of postoperative vomiting.

Adult doses: 0.2–0.4 mg IM, 8 hourly;
     300 µg oral, 6 hourly.

Transdermal preparation—this releases approximately 500 µg in 72 h and should be applied to a hairless area of skin behind the ear.

Butyrophenone derivatives

These are centrally acting dopamine antagonist drugs with specific effects upon the chemoreceptor trigger zone. They also have sedative effects and unwanted extrapyramidal effects are also seen.

Droperidol

This drug is widely used in anaesthesia in combination with opioid drugs for its sedative effects. In low doses it is a good antiemetic following surgery.

Adult doses: 2.5–5 mg IV, 6 hourly;
     2.5–5 mg IM, 6 hourly;
     5 mg oral, 4–8 hourly.

Paediatrics: 0.5–1 mg daily in divided doses IM or oral.

For vomiting associated with cancer chemotherapy, doses of 20–75 µg/kg IM or IV may be required.

Other dopamine antagonists

Metoclopramide

This drug has central actions closely resembling the phenothiazine antiemetics. In addition, it has peripheral actions upon the gastrointestinal tract. These include an increase in the tone of the lower oesophageal sphincter and increased rate of gastric emptying. The peripheral actions of metoclopramide are antagonized by atropine administration. Extrapyramidal side-effects also occur and are seen most frequently in young female patients.

Adult doses:	5–10 mg IV, 8 hourly;	
	5–10 mg IM, 6–8 hourly;	
	10 mg oral, 8 hourly.	
Paediatrics:	< 1 year	1 mg, 12 hourly;
	1–3 years	1 mg, 8–12 hourly;
	3–5 years	2 mg, 8–12 hourly;
	5–9 years	2.5 mg, 8–12 hourly;
	9–14 years	5 mg, 8–12 hourly.

Domperidone

This agent does not readily cross the blood–brain barrier and so is less likely to produce central side-effects such as sedation and acute dystonic reactions. It is an effective antiemetic and is often used in the treatment of nausea and vomiting associated with cytotoxic chemotherapy.

Adult doses:	10–20 mg oral, 4–8 hourly;
	60 mg suppository, 4–8 hourly.
Paediatrics:	200–400 μg/kg oral.

Alternative therapies

Acupuncture

Traditional Chinese acupuncture techniques have been investigated in the management of postoperative nausea and vomiting and found to be effective. The acupuncture point is known as *Nei-kuan* and is located 5 cm proximal to the most distal wrist crease, between the tendons of palmaris longus and flexor carpi radialis on the right forearm. The needle should be inserted perpendicular to the skin to a depth of approximately 1.5–2.5 cm. Electric stimulation with low current—electro acupuncture—can be applied to the needle.

Acupressure

This is an alternative where bands maintaining pressure over this position can be worn around the wrist. They have been useful for motion sickness in children but are not effective in postoperative nausea and vomiting.

17 Case studies in pain management

The patient studies in this chapter have been chosen to illustrate commonly encountered problems in the accident and emergency department as well as those in the medical and surgical wards.

Techniques such as regional blockade and the administration of epidural opioids may not be widely available and staff should seek help if unsure about the practice in their particular unit.

In all instances it is important to maintain attention to the patient's general condition and specifically to ensure an adequate airway, oxygenation, and the correction of hypovolaemia or other cause of shock in the individual patient, as necessary.

Major postoperative pain

> *A 53 year old man has undergone a surgical procedure for repair of a hiatus hernia. The operation was performed through an upper abdominal incision extended into a left thoractomy.*

This example is characteristic of a patient who has undergone major upper-abdominal or thoracic surgery. Pain control following such procedures can be achieved by a number of methods.

Option 1: opioids

At the present time opioid drugs remain the mainstay of management of such patients. Acute severe pain immediately postoperatively will require parenteral therapy. Intravenous bolus doses of morphine—5 mg, for one or two doses, followed by 2.5 mg given as often as necessary to control the patient's pain and titrated to the patient's response. An interval of 2–3 min should be allowed between doses to allow the morphine to diffuse into the brain and exert its effects.

Intravenous infusions of opioids are commonly used in this group of patients (see Chapter 9), papaveretum or morphine being most commonly used. Bolus doses of morhpine (5 mg followed by 2.5 mg increments) should be administered to gain early control of the pain and then an infusion of morphine commenced at a rate of 3–5 mg/h. The recurrence of pain during the infusion may be controlled by further small bolus doses (2.5 mg) and the rate increased. The infusion rate should be maintained at the lowest rate consistent with good analgesia and the patient's general condition and pain control assessed frequently.

If available, the use of patient-controlled analgesia systems with intravenous opioids is a useful alternative.

Option 2: the epidural route

This route, using local anaesthetic agents or opioids, is gaining increasing favour as the method of choice for analgesia in these patients. The insertion of catheters into the epidural space is most often performed immediately preoperatively by the anaesthetist. It offers intraoperative analgesia as well as continuing analgesia during the early postoperative period. Useful analgesia has been obtained with morphine and fentanyl alone or in combination with local anaesthetic agents. Local anaesthetic agents, however, are likely to produce sympathetic blockade, which may potentiate hypotension in the hypovolaemic patient. Epidural analgesia may be provided by continuous infusions via the epidural catheter or repeated bolus doses may be given.

For upper-abdominal surgery the catheter should be sited in the lower thoracic region. A bolus dose of 5 ml of 0.5 per cent bupivacaine is administered and the extent of analgesia can be checked by loss of sensation to pinprick over the thoracic dermatomes. Infusions of local anaesthetic agents may be used and an appropriate rate would be 3–7 ml of 0.25 per cent bupivacaine per hour. If infusions are used the extent of the block should be checked regularly. Because of the hazards of local anaesthetic agents the patient must be in a high dependency unit.

Opioid drugs administered by the epidural route include morphine and fentanyl (see Chapter 11). An appropriate dose would be morphine 2 mg, repeated eight-hourly if necessary.

Option 3: local anaesthetic techniques
(See Chapter 14).

Intercostal nerve blocks   An alternative local anaesthetic technique is the use of intercostal nerve blocks. This avoids the effects of sympathetic blockade, provides good analgesia, but may require multiple injections causing discomfort to the patient. There is a small risk of pneumothorax from the procedure. The first blocks may be performed intraoperatively by the surgeon before chest closure, providing analgesia in the early postoperative period.

Interpleural analgesia   Interpleural injection of local anaesthetic is a recent development; bupivacaine is the most commonly used local anaesthetic and is administered via a catheter inserted between the parietal and visceral pleura (p. 116); 20 ml of 0.5 per cent bupivacaine is injected through the catheter and this may be repeated at four- to six-hourly intervals.

Major trauma

> *A 24 year old man was admitted to hospital after a road traffic accident. He was the front seat passenger in a car involved in a head-on collision. On assessment in Casualty he has fractured the 6th to 10th ribs on the left, has fractures of his left tibia and left forearm, and is deeply unconscious. He has scalp lacerations and is bleeding from his nose and left ear.*

The undesirable side effects of parenteral analgesics may present a hazard to the multiply-injured trauma patient. Particular problems may be associated with

(1) respiratory depression;

(2) depression of the cough reflex;

(3) depression of conscious level;

(4) hypotension;

If there are concerns about any of these then expert help and advice should be obtained.

However, alleviating pain and discomfort is an important goal of early management of trauma patients. The effects of pain control must therefore be closely monitored for efficacy and adverse effects.

This patient has a serious head injury. If respiratory depression from opioid administration occurs then the associated increase in the arterial partial pressure of carbon dioxide will increase cerebral blood flow. This, in turn, may cause a significant increase in intracranial pressure, worsening the head injury. There is no place in this patient for epidural techniques, which may also cause elevation of intracranial pressure or exacerbate any hypotension due to hypovolaemia.

In this patient anaesthetic assistance should be urgently sought and intermittent positive-pressure ventilation should be instituted rapidly. This ensures adequate oxygenation and ventilation. Hyperventilation and the resulting low $PaCO_2$ will aid in the reduction of intracranial pressure. Opioids may then be used to facilitate mechanical control of ventilation. Morphine in 2.5 mg boluses, fentanyl 100 μg, or phenoperidine 1 mg boluses may be given along with non-depolarizing muscle-relaxant drugs.

The chest injury in this patient (pulmonary contusion, flail segments, and possible aspiration) may also benefit from mechanical ventilation and the respiratory depressant and antitussive effects of the opioids are then useful.

Limb fractures

An 18 year old female is admitted with a fractured shaft of femur after a fall from a horse.

It is important to note that early stabilization and immobilization of limb fractures will reduce pain. The severity of pain in the affected limb may be aggravated by spasm in muscle groups around the fracture site. Regional anaesthesia producing muscle relaxation will benefit this patient. The provision of good pain relief in the Accident and Emergency department is important.

This patient will be subjected to numerous examinations and may need to be moved and X-rayed many times, all of which increase pain, discomfort, and distress.

Whenever a limb fracture occurs, care should be taken to observe the vascular state of the limb. Ischaemia developing in fractured limbs is normally extremely painful. This pain may be abolished with the analgesia produced from regional blockade.

The most suitable technique to provide analgesia in this patient is a femoral nerve block. Where staff skilled in regional anaesthetic techniques are not available, alternative analgesia must be provided by the parenteral administration of opioid drugs. Initially the pain may be controlled by intravenous bolus doses of morphine 2.5–5 mg, with further intermittent bolus doses parenterally to maintain analgesia until the fractured femur is stabilized.

Rib fractures

> *A 23 year old man is admitted to hospital after a fall from scaffolding. He has fractures of his right 5th, 6th, and 7th ribs. The pain restricts his breathing and he develops progressive pulmonary collapse and consolidation.*

Multiple fractured ribs are often associated with other injuries, usually after major trauma, and these must be excluded. The problems from the chest injury result from both the alteration of chest-wall mechanics and from underlying pulmonary contusion caused by the injury. Reduction in the chest-wall compliance after rib fractures leads to an increase in the work of breathing, tidal volumes are reduced, gas exchange is impaired, and atelectasis and pneumonia develop. Analgesia should therefore restore pulmonary function and avoid respiratory depression.

Effective therapies include the following.

Intercostal nerve blockade
This should include blockade of the fourth to eighth intercostal nerves (see p. 114): 3 ml of bupivacaine 0.5 per cent with

adrenalin should be injected at each intercostal space. Blocks may need to be performed more posteriorly (p. 116). The injections may need to be repeated eight-hourly.

Epidural local anaesthetics and opioids (p. 121)
The insertion of a thoracic epidural catheter requires the assistance of an anaesthetist and therefore this technique may not always be an available option. Doses of local anaesthetics and opioids administered via the epidural route would be similar to those described for the first patient in this section.

Interpleural local anaesthetic administration (p. 116)
If a pneumothorax is present in association with the rib fractures the local anaesthetic may be instilled through the chest drain.

Patient-controlled opioid analgesia
The use of patient-controlled systems to deliver intravenous opioids will be useful if these systems are available.

Renal colic

> *A 35 year old man presents with severe right-sided loin pain of sudden onset, radiating to the groin. He gives a history of a previous episode of similar pain associated with a ureteric calculus, which was passed spontaneously.*

The stretching of the ureteral muscle as the ureter contracts around the stone during peristalsis causes ischaemia which results in pain. It is referred through the lower thoracic (T11 and T12) and lumbar (L1) nerves. Hyperalgesia in the cutaneous distribution of these nerves may also be felt.

As for the management of all acute pain the requirements of analgesia for this patient include a rapid onset of analgesia and minimal circulatory disturbance. A low incidence of nausea and vomiting is desirable to allow the patient to drink freely, a high fluid input being maintained to prevent further stone formation. In addition the effects of the analgesic drug used upon the smooth muscle of the ureter is important. Maintenance of ureteric peristalsis will increase the likelihood of the calculus being passed spontaneously. The effects of opioids on smooth muscle, increasing tone and spasm, may be a disadvantage in this patient. Pethidine, 75–100 mg IM, or 25 mg IV repeated as necessary to bring the pain under control, is generally regarded as the opioid of choice. Although it does increase smooth-muscle spasm, this effect is less than that produced by morphine. As a result of the adverse effects of opioids, parenteral NSAIDs have become the analgesics of choice. A suitable regime with diclofenac is 75 mg IM with a further 75 mg IM after 30 min if necessary.

Myocardial pain

> *A 58 year old man is admitted with severe central-chest pain radiating to the neck and left arm. He has a history of angina on exertion but this pain is unrelated to exercise and has not been relieved by nitrates.*

The classical pain of myocardial ischaemia is central chest pain, retrosternal, radiating to the neck, jaw, and left arm. It may be improved by therapy aimed at improving myocardial perfusion such as nitrates, vasodilator drugs, or thrombolytic agents. Prolonged pain may be associated with crescendo angina or myocardial infarction. Analgesic agents used in this situation should have minimal cardiovascular-depressant effects. The common opioids used are morphine (5–10 mg) or diamorphine (5 mg) given intravenously. Other opioids that have been shown to be suitable are meptazinol (100 mg), nalbuphine (10 mg), and buprenorphine (0.3 mg). The pain associated with myocardial infarction will generally only require one or two doses of parenteral opioid.

Burns

> *A 45 year old woman is admitted following a house fire. She has 15–20 per cent burns, mainly around her arms and upper body. There is no evidence of smoke inhalation or airway burns.*

In the early stage following severe burns, pain may be a relatively minor problem. Full thickness and deep partial thickness burns are painless. However, pain control over prolonged periods may be necessary in burned patients and may need flexibility to cover the pain and distress of debridement of wounds and dressing changes.

Intravenous opioids such as morphine 2.5–5 mg should be given initially to control the pain. If frequent doses are required (every 30–40 min) then an infusion of morphine, starting at 5 mg per hour and adjusting the rate up or down as necessary, may be helpful. PCA systems have been used successfully for parenteral opioid administration. Children with burns also benefit from cognitive and behavioural regimes used in addition to opioid drugs to achieve better pain relief.

18 Pain control in special situations

Obstetrics

Analgesia for the obstetric patient is unusual in that the doctor must consider two patients—the fetus and the mother—and the effects the chosen method of analgesia will have on both. It is also a situation in which the patients themselves may express a preference for particular methods of analgesia.

Analgesia may be required for labour, following operative procedures performed during pregnancy such as cervical cerclage (Shirodkar suture), and after Caesarian section.

Pain relief in labour is a major topic and, other than a brief review, is beyond the scope of this book. Interested readers are referred to the additional reading lists for this chapter.

Psychological preparation

Psychological and behavioural methods have been widely used in preparation for, and to alleviate the pain of, labour for many centuries. Hypnosis has been used at intervals since it was first described by Mesmer in 1777. Current methods involve relaxation and dissociation techniques, which are taught during pregnancy in preparation for labour.

Sedatives and analgesics

Methods of analgesia have changed over the centuries with the development of potent analgesic and anaesthetic agents. Ether was the first inhalational agent and was used in 1847. Analgesia for labour achieved respect following the administration of chloroform 'à la reine' after providing analgesia for the birth of Queen Victoria's eighth child in 1853. Inhalational techniques remain popular today—using a nitrous oxide/oxygen mixture—Entonox (see Chapter 15).

Combinations of opioid drugs and sedatives were popular in the first half of the 20th century, particularly the use of morphine and papaveretum with sedatives such as barbiturates or hyoscine. In recent times, pethidine and newer synthetic opioids such as meptazinol have replaced these agents as the standard systemic analgesics.

Regional anaesthetic techniques

Epidural analgesia with local anaesthetic agents is well established for providing good analgesia during labour and anaesthesia for operative obstetric procedures. Analgesia during labour may be provided by intermittent bolus doses of local anaesthetics, of which bupivacaine is the agent most frequently used, and these 'top-up' doses may be administered by trained midwives. Continuous infusions of local anaesthetic solutions into the epidural space provides improved analgesia, and once the block is established there will be continuous analgesia without intermittent episodes of pain that can occur between top-ups. More recently the combination of opioid drugs with local anaesthetic agents administered into the epidural space has been used to produce analgesia for labour and also for postoperative pain control. Epidural opioids will reduce the requirements for further local anaesthetic administration via the epidural route during labour. They may also result in improved perineal analgesia during labour.

Transcutaneous nerve stimulation (TENS)

The analgesia provided by continuous painless stimuli applied in the region of a painful stimulus has been interpreted as a 'closing of the gate' to transmission of pain at the spinal cord level (see Chapter 2). When used to provide analgesia in labour, external electrical stimulation from two pairs of electrodes attached to either side of the spine in the thoraco-lumbar and sacral regions is used. A low-intensity stimulus is applied continuously with a higher intensity applied during contractions only. Its use is generally helpful in the first stage of labour and allows the mother to remain mobile. It is also acceptable to those women who are reluctant to accept pharmacological methods of pain control in labour.

Ideal analgesia for labour

Any techniques used during labour should produce efficient relief from pain whilst maintaining consciousness between contractions and good patient co-operation. It should not influence the process of labour. Respiratory depression, particularly of the neonate, should be minimal.

The advantages and disadvantages of analgesic techniques during labour

Systemic opioid administration still remains the most common method of analgesia in labour although it has significant adverse effects. The most important of these is neonatal respiratory depression. This results from placental transfer of the opioid drugs from the mother to the fetus. Delayed elimination in the newborn infant, due to immature renal and hepatic function, can prolong these effects and necessitate the use of naloxone. Opioids delay gastric emptying in the mother. This is a major risk factor if an operative procedure is required, since stomach contents can be vomited or regurgitated during general anaesthesia, resulting in pulmonary aspiration. This complication carries a high mortality.

Patients may dislike opioid analgesia because of the drowsiness, nausea, and vomiting associated with opioid administration. The indeterminate length of labour may lead to inadequate provision of analgesia by this method. A patient requesting analgesia who is given an intramuscular injection of opioid and then delivers rapidly may have very little benefit, since drug absorption may not be sufficiently rapid to achieve good analgesia. Such patients may obtain better analgesia from the use of an intravenous opioid.

PCA systems have also been used to administer intravenous opioids on demand during labour, although they have not found widespread acceptance for this use. They are also used to provide postoperative analgesia after Caesarian section.

Regional techniques such as epidural and spinal blocks require technical expertise and a readily available anaesthetist. They also require increased observations of the patient by the midwifery staff once the epidural is sited, and designated staff must be responsible for the administration of repeated bolus doses to maintain analgesia. In some patients, epidural techniques will fail to provide adequate analgesia with localized areas remaining without analgesia (missed segment) or even one side with no analgesia (unilateral block). The sympathetic block, associated with epidural local anaesthetic administration, may result in profound hypotension. This may be exacerbated by the aortocaval compression which occurs when the pregnant patient is supine. When this occurs the gravid uterus compresses the inferior vena cava. This reduces venous return which in turn results in a decrease in cardiac output and hypotension. It is therefore important to turn the patient on to her side to prevent this. Motor blockade is a further disadvantage when there is a need to retain patient mobility and ability to 'push' in the second stage of labour.

Inadvertent intravascular administration of local anaesthetic agent may occur after epidural administration, resulting in systemic toxicity. This may occur if the catheter is incorrectly placed initially or it may be delayed, and associated with subsequent top-up doses, if the catheter erodes into a vein at a later stage. Intrathecal administration may occur after a bolus dose through the epidural cannula resulting in a high block with hypotension and respiratory difficulty. This may occur with the initial dose of local anaesthetic if the catheter has been sited intradurally or with later top-ups if the catheter erodes through the dura. These dangerous sequelae are rare.

Dural puncture with the large 16 G Tuohy needle may occur during the siting of an epidural. It may be associated with a distressing post-lumbar-puncture headache which can interfere with the ability of the mother to care for her infant and may require an 'epidural blood patch' to improve the symptoms (see p. 127).

Postoperative analgesia

When Caesarian section has been performed under regional block, postoperative analgesia may be continued by epidural opioids. After general anaesthesia, PCA systems and intravenous opioid infusions are useful.

Opioid drugs are excreted in breast milk, although the amounts that are present after conventional analgesic regimes are unlikely to produce adverse effects in the neonate.

PAEDIATRICS

The control of acute pain in children has been poorly investigated. However, when information is available, it shows that pain control is rarely satisfactory.

Little information has been available about pain perception and response in infants and children. Early work suggested that pain perception was not established until about three months of age. This was believed to be a result of the incomplete myelination present at birth. More recent studies have shown clear evidence of cardiorespiratory and hormonal responses to pain, demonstrating that neonates do respond to pain. Variations in sensitivity to pain have not been investigated in older infants and children although it has been suggested that pain thresholds may increase with age. However, it is often observed that younger children will return to play more quickly after painful procedures and are perceived as having less pain than older children after equivalent operations. In direct comparison to adults with similarly painful conditions, children receive considerably less analgesia even after cardiac surgery.

Problems may arise in the management of pain in children as a result of the following.

1. Increased sensitivity of very young children, particularly premature infants, to the depressant effects of opioid drugs. Infants under three months of age should not be given opioids unless in a carefully monitored environment such as an intensive care unit or neonatal unit where respiratory monitoring is available and there are facilities for ventilatory support if necessary. Infants who are between three and six months of age may have no greater respiratory depression from opioids than adults although most would prescribe smaller doses of opioid drugs for this age group.

2. Assessment of pain in children can be difficult. In the pre-verbal infant, attempts to correlate crying frequencies to painful stimuli have not been successful, although characteristic facial expressions that can be associated with painful stimulations may prove to be a useful measure in the very young infant. In older children, from about three years of age, the concept of 'hurt' and

that there are varying degrees of it is understood. However, children of this age group find it difficult to express the level of their 'hurt' unless appropriate devices such as picture scales or rungs on a ladder are available to help.

3. Nursing staff may show a reluctance about using intra-muscular injections for pain control. Children may find injections painful and unpleasant and be reticent about asking for analgesia as a consequence.

4. Care must be taken over the calculation of doses for children and then in the administration of the correct doses. This may involve several dilutions of the original presentation or the administration of very small volumes of concentrated drug, which can produce errors. Doses may be calculated in terms of body weight or surface area.

Aids to the assessment of pain in children

Direct communication

- *Verbalization*—what the child actually says about his/her pain. Self-report scales are the most reliable method of assessment but children must learn how to use them. Listening to the child's description and accepting the level described is important. Criticism of the child and comments such as 'is the pain really that bad?' from adults will make the child agree with the adult.

- *Vocalization*—non-specific crying or whining features.

- *Body language*—pointing to or guarding the painful area.

Indirect, behavioural methods

- *Activity*—a child in pain will be reluctant to move or play.

- *Appearance*—pallor and sweating may be associated with pain.

- *Temperament*—pain is unpleasant and the child may be miserable, withdrawn, and unco-operative. Some children may respond to pain with aggressive behaviour.

- *Interactions with others*—pain may make the child fearful and they may then not respond to surroundings or people, preferring to be close to parents, with whom they feel secure.

Physiological status

Pain is associated with increased levels of circulating catecholamines. These will produce characteristic physiological changes, which can be used as objective measures of pain. Such monitoring could include

- pulse rate—increases with pain;
- blood pressure—also increases with pain.

Sweating and pallor may be seen.

Changes with time

It is important to monitor the effect of analgesics over a period of time to ensure that relief from pain is obtained both initially and during recovery. Other features such as nausea, tiredness, and uncomfortable positions, as well as psychological factors such as fear and anxiety, can make a child's pain feel worse. These should be noted and managed appropriately.

Suggestions for improvements in paediatric pain control

1. Greater use of local anaesthetic techniques in the intra-operative period to provide postoperative analgesia, for example wound infiltration, caudal epidural blocks, or nerve blocks. These add little extra time to the operation but provide great benefit after recovery from anaesthesia. Local anaesthetic procedures may be performed during general anaesthesia, then any discomfort which would be felt by an awake child will be avoided.

2. Continuous intravenous infusions of opioid analgesics will reduce the need for unpleasant intramuscular injections and improve postoperative pain relief. The siting of an intravenous cannula can be performed while the child is anaesthetized, when discomfort for the child will be avoided and venous access may be facilitated by the dilatation of veins produced by volatile anaesthetics such as halothane or isoflurane. It is preferable to maintain a separate intravenous infusion site for the opioid infusion (see Chapters 9 and 10); sequestration of analgesic within intravenous fluids administered through the same cannula can lead to an overdose of analgesic if these other fluids are administered rapidly.

The use of morphine by continuous intravenous infusion to provide good analgesia following major surgery (abdominal and thoracic) in children has been described by Bray (1983). A modified regime is described below:

> body weight (kg) $\times$ ½ = milligrams of morphine;
> make up to 50 ml in a syringe pump;
> infusion rate 1–2 ml/h.

3. Children may also use patient-controlled analgesia (see Chapter 10). More recently there has been a trend towards the use of parent- and patient-controlled analgesia or parent-assisted analgesia. In this situation the parent, who is staying in the same room as the child, is also instructed in the use of the PCA system and may make demands to improve the pain control as well as the child. In early reports most parents have found this useful, although others have expressed anxiety about being in charge of the system. No problems have been reported and good analgesia is achieved with this technique.

Psychological techniques

Children respond particularly well to psychological interventions (Chapter 4). Reinforcement techniques, where the child is rewarded for positive behaviours and coping with the pain, whereas negative behaviour such as moaning, complaining, or avoidance of activity is ignored, have been used in situations where there is excessive pain behaviour. Treatments that seek to change the level of attention to, or perception of, the pain, including hypnosis and cognitive coping strategies such as distraction and dissociation are also helpful. Biofeedback and relaxation techniques may also be useful for painful procedures such as venepuncture in the older child who is afraid of needles.

The important concept that children suffer pain and that it may require aggressive treatment is only the beginning of improving pain control in children. The differences between children and adults in the expression of pain and the differing requirements for treatment are important. Careful consideration must be given to the child's developmental stage when monitoring the response to pain and analgesia. The wider use of additional techniques, the greater numbers of interested staff available, and future research may hopefully improve the management of acute pain in children.

PROBLEM PATIENTS

Geriatrics

The elderly patient shows increased drug sensitivity. Clearance of many drugs is reduced with increasing age because of age-related decreases in both renal and hepatic function. These features explain the need to increase the time interval between analgesic drug doses in the elderly. For example, morphine may be administered at six-hourly intervals to a 90 year old patient, whilst in a fit 18 year old, even three-hourly administration may be insufficient.

The use of standard analgesic doses in the elderly population may result in the increased incidence of adverse effects.

Many elderly patients have coexisting medical problems which must be taken into consideration when prescribing analgesia. For example, cardiovascular function may be impaired and congestive cardiac failure may result from the use of NSAIDs as a result of fluid retention. In addition, patients with chronic obstructive airways disease may be at increased risk from the respiratory-depressant effects of opioid drugs.

Increasing use of local and regional analgesic techniques after major surgery and trauma will be beneficial in this group of patients.

Critically ill patients

It is often difficult to obtain good pain control in these patients while avoiding unwanted effects of the drugs. Factors which may contribute to the problems include the following.

1. There may be difficulty in assessing pain, which may remain unrecognized, in a sedated, paralysed patient receiving mechanical ventilation.
2. Altered drug sensitivity in the critically ill patients may result in greater adverse effects.

3. Reduced hepatic or renal function will delay metabolism and excretion of drugs. Toxic effects may result from the accumulation of the drugs themselves, or from the action of metabolites.

4. Drug interactions will also be of importance in this group who may be receiving large numbers of drugs during their stay in the intensive care unit.

5. Critically ill patients may require treatment for prolonged periods and drug accumulation and side-effects are therefore more likely.

6. The respiratory-depressant effects of opioids may hinder weaning of patients from mechanical ventilation, adversely affecting their recovery.

7. Careful titration of dose and regular assessment of the effect of drugs are essential. Some patients may benefit from the use of regional analgesia. Epidural techniques using opioids or local anaesthetics may be useful for prolonged analgesia in suitable patients. Patient- or nurse-controlled analgesia delivery systems may also be helpful in this group of patients.

PAIN SPECIALISTS

Pain clinics have been developed over many years in response to the needs of patients principally with chronic pain. More recently, particularly in the USA, acute pain specialists have been responding to the need for improvement in the overall management of acute pain in hospitals.

The aim of an acute pain service is to provide expert assistance from trained staff, medical and nursing, with access to more techniques and equipment appropriate to the needs of patients with acute pain. In addition, the service aims to improve the level of knowledge of staff caring for patients with acute pain.

The wealth of evidence documenting the poor treatment of acute pain would suggest that this service will be beneficial in increasing patient comfort and satisfaction during their hospital stay.

At present, help in the management of pain which is difficult to control will usually be available from the members of staff of intensive care units, anaesthetic departments, or pain clinics. In addition, the assistance of allied specialists including psycho-therapists, psychiatrists, and pharmacologists may be helpful in improving pain management and in stimulating research.

Suggested additional reading

CHAPTERS 1-5

BEECHER, H.K. (1956a). Relationship of significance of wound to pain experienced. *Journal of the American Medical Association*, 161, 1609-13.

BEECHER, H.K. (1956b). The subjective response and reaction to sensation. *American Journal of Medicine*, 20, 107-13.

BUDD, K. (1989). Pain: theory and management. In *Scientific Foundations of anaesthesia* (ed. C. Scurr, S. Feldman, and N. Soni). Heinemann Medical, Oxford.

CHAPMAN, C.R. (1989). *Assessment of pain in anaesthesia* (ed. W.S. Nimmo and G. Smith). Blackwell Scientific Publications, Oxford.

CHAPMAN, C.R., CASEY, K.L., DUBNER, R., FOLEY, K.M., GRACELY, R.H., and READING, A.E. (1985). Pain measurement: an overview. *Pain*, 2, 1-31.

DODSON, M.E. (ed.) (1985). The management of postoperative pain. *Current topics in anaesthesia, Vol. 8*. Edward Arnold, London.

DUTHIE, D.J.R. (1989). *The physiology and pharmacology of pain in anaesthesia* (ed. W. S. Nimmo and G. Smith). Blackwell Scientific Publications, Oxford.

EGAN, K.J. (1989). Psychological issues in postoperative pain in management of postoperative pain. *Anesthesiology Clinics of North America*, 7, 183-92.

FERNANDEZ, E. (1986). A classification system of cognitive coping strategies for pain. *Pain*, 26, 141-51.

KEHLET, H. (1989). Surgical stress: the role of pain and analgesia. *British Journal of Anaesthesia*, 63, 189-95.

MANN, R.D. (ed.) (1988). *The history of the management of pain—from early principles to present practice*. Parthenon, Carnforth Lancs.

MELZACK, R. and WALL, P.D. (1965). Pain mechanisms: a new theory. *Science*, 150, 971-9.

NAYMAN, J. (1979). Measurement and control of postoperative pain. *Annals of the Royal College of Surgeons of England*, 61, 419-26.

OTTOSON, D. (1983). *Physiology of the nervous system*. Macmillan, London.

PORTER, J. and JICK, H. (1980). Addiction rare in patients treated with narcotics. *New England Journal of Medicine*, 302, 123.

REMETZ, M.S. and CABIN, H.S. (1988). Analgesic therapy in acute myocardial infarction. *Cardiology Clinics*, 6, 29-36.

TAENZER, P., MELZACK, R., and JEANS, M.E. (1986). Influence of psychological factors on postoperative pain, mood and analgesic requirements. *Pain*, 24, 331-42.

SPENCER, R.T. (1989). Drug therapy for pain relief. In: *Clinical pharmacology and nursing management* (3rd edn), (ed. R.T. Spencer, L.W. Nichols, G.B. Lipkin, H.M. Sabo, and F.M. West). J.B. Lippincott Co., Philadelphia.

WALL, P.D. (1980). The role of the substantia gelatinosa as a gate control. In *Pain* (ed. J.J. Bonica). Raven Press, New York.

WILKIE, D.J., HOLZEMER, W.L., TESLER, M.D. *et al.* (1990). Measuring pain quality: validity and reliability of children's and adolescent's pain language. *Pain*, 41, 151-9.

ZIMMERMAN, M. (1979). Peripheral and central nervous mechanisms of nociception, pain and pain therapy. In *Advances in pain research and therapy* (ed. J.J. Bonica). Raven Press, New York.

CHAPTER 6

BENET, L.Z. and SHEINER, L.B. (1985). Pharmacokinetics: The dynamics of drug absorption, distribution, and elimination. In *The pharmacological basis of therapeutics* (ed. A.G. Gilman, L.S. Goodman, T.W. Rall, and F. Murad). Macmillan, London.

MATHER, L.E. (1983). Pharmacokinetic and pharmacodynamic factors influencing the choice, dose and route of administration of opiates for acute pain. *Clinics in Anesthesiology*, 1, 17-40.

CHAPTERS 7 AND 8

BULLINGHAM, R.E.S. (ed.) (1983). Opiate analgesia. *Clinics in Anesthesiology*, 1, 1. Saunders, London.

DUTHIE, D.J.R. and NIMMO, W.S. (1987). Adverse effects of opioid analgesic drugs. *British Journal of Anaesthesia*, 59, 61-77.

FREYE, E. (1987). *Opioid agonists, antagonists and mixed narcotic analgesics: theoretical background and considerations for practical use*. Springer, Berlin.

HUG, C.C. (1984). Pharmacokinetics and pharmacodynamics of narcotic analgesics. In *Pharmacokinetics of anaesthesia* (ed. C. Prys-Roberts and C.C. Hug, Jr). Blackwell Scientific Publications, Oxford.

JAFFE, J.H. and MARTIN, W.R. (1985). Opioid analgesics and antagonists. In *The pharmacological basis of therapeutics* (ed. A.G. Gilman, L.S. Goodman, T.W. Rall, and F. Murad). Macmillan, London.

CHAPTER 9

HULL, C.J. (1985). Opioid infusions for the management of post-operative pain. In *Acute pain* (ed. G. Smith and B.G. Covino). Butterworth, London.

CHAPTER 10

FERRANTE, F.M., OSTHEIMER, G.W., and COVINO, B.G. (ed.) (1990). *Patient controlled analgesia* (2nd edn). Blackwell Scientific Publications, Oxford.

HARMER, M., ROSEN, M., and VICKERS, M.D. (ed.) (1985). *Patient controlled analgesia*. Blackwell Scientific Publications, Oxford.

MATHER, L.E. and OWEN, H. (1988). The scientific basis of patient-controlled analgesia. *Anaesthesia and Intensive Care*, 16, 427-37.

OWEN, H., MATHER, L.E., and ROWLEY, K. (1988). The development and clinical use of patient-controlled analgesia. *Anaesthesia and Intensive Care*, 16, 437-47.

WHITE, P.F. (1988). Use of patient controlled analgesia for management of acute pain. *Journal of the American Medical Association*, 259, 243-7.

CHAPTER 11

COUSINS, M.J. and MATHER, L.E. (1984). Intrathecal and epidural administration of opioids. *Anesthesiology*, 61, 276-310.

MORGAN, M. (1989). The rational use of intrathecal and extradural opioids. *British Journal of Anaesthesia*, 63, 165-88.

CHAPTERS 13 AND 14

COUSINS, M.J. and BRIDENBAUGH, P.O. (ed.) (1980). *Neural blockade in clinical anesthesia and management of pain*. J.B. Lippincott Co., Philadelphia.

DALENS, B. (1989). Regional anesthesia in children. *Anesthesia and Analgesia*, 68, 654-72.

ERIKSSON, E. (1979). *Illustrated handbook in local anaesthesia* (2nd edn). Lloyd-Luke (Medical Books) Ltd, London.

REYNOLDS, F. (1987). Adverse effects of local anaesthetics. *British Journal of Anaesthesia*, 59, 78-95.

SCOTT, D.B., McCLURE, J., and WILDSMITH, J.A.W. (ed.) (1984). *Regional anaesthesia 1884-1984*, Centennial Meeting of Regional Anaesthesia, Information Consulting Medical, Södertälje, Sweden.

SCOTT, D.B. (1989). *Techniques of regional anaesthesia*. Appleton and Lange/Mediglobe, and Prentice-Hall, New York.

CHAPTER 15

FINCK, A.D. (1985). Nitrous oxide analgesia. In *Nitrous oxide* (ed. E.I. Eger II). Edward Arnold, London.

CHAPTER 16

GILLIES, H.C., ROGERS, H.J., SPECTOR, R.G., and TROUNCE, J.R. (1986). *A textbook of clinical pharmacology*. Hodder and Stoughton, London.

GRAHAME-SMITH, D.G. (1986). Vomiting and anti-emetic therapy. In *Topics in gastroenterology* Vol. 14. (ed. D.P. Jewell and A. Ireland). Blackwell Scientific Publications, Oxford.

LAURENCE, D.R., BENNETT, R.N. (1987). *Clinical pharmacology*. Churchill Livingstone, London.

CHAPTER 18

Obstetrics

CRAWFORD, J.S. (1982). *Obstetric analgesia and anaesthesia*. Churchill Livingstone, Edinburgh.

MOIR, D.D. and THORBURN, J. (1986). Obstetric anaesthesia and analgesia (3rd edn). Baillière Tindall, Eastbourne.

MORGAN, B.M. (1987). Analgesia in labour. In *Foundations of obstetric anaesthesia* (ed. B.M. Morgan). Farrand Press, London.

Paediatrics

BERDE, C.B. (1989). Pediatric postoperative pain management. *Pediatric Clinics of North America—Acute Pain in Children*, 36, 921-39.

BRAY, R.J. (1983). Postoperative analgesia provided by morphine infusion in children. *Anaesthesia*, **38**, 1075-8.

LLOYD-THOMAS, A.R. (1990). Pain management in paediatric patients. *British Journal of Anaesthesia*, **64**, 85-104.

MCGRATH, P.J. and CRAIG, K.D. (1989). Developmental and psychological factors in children's pain. *Pediatric clinics of North America—Acute Pain in Children*, **36**, 823-36.

SCHECHTER, N.L. (1989). The undertreatment of pain in children: an overview. *Pediatric Clinics of North America—Acute Pain in Children*, **36**, 781-94.

THOMPSON, K.L. and VARNI, J.W. (1986). A developmental cognitive-biobehavioural approach to pediatric pain assessment. *Pain*, **25**, 283-96.

Index